Drugs and People

Medications, Their History and Origins, and the Way They Act

Drugs and People

Medications, Their History and Origins, and the Way They Act

REVISED EDITION

ALFRED BURGER

UNIVERSITY PRESS OF VIRGINIA
Charlottesville

THE UNIVERSITY PRESS OF VIRGINIA

First published 1986. Revised edition 1988

LIBRARY OF CONGRESS
Library of Congress Cataloging-in-Publication Data

Burger, Alfred, 1905-
Drugs and people : medications, their history and origins, and the way they act / Alfred Burger. -- Rev. ed.
p. cm.
Includes index.
1. Pharmacology--Popular works. 2. Drugs. 3. Drugs--History.
I. Title.
RM301.15.B87 1988
615'.1--dc19 88-12218
CIP

ISBN 0-8139-1101-X

Notice Concerning Patent or Trade Mark Rights. The listing or discussion in this book of any drug in respect to which patent or trade mark rights may exist shall not be deemed, and is not intended as, a grant of, or authority to exercise, or an infringement of, any right or privilege protected by such patent or trade mark.

Printed in the United States of America

Contents

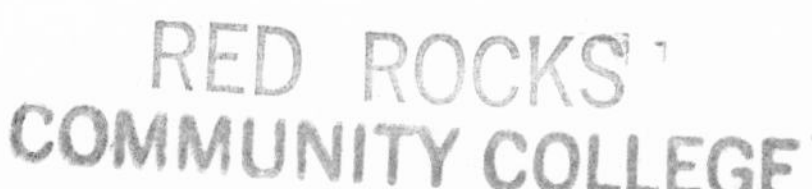

Preface

This book is for persons who are interested in medicines and who want to know where drugs come from, how they were discovered or conceived, and what drugs do after they enter the body. No profound knowledge of chemistry or other sciences will be required because the language is simple and whenever technical words are needed they are explained in plain English. Some accounts in this book are not precise enough to satisfy the professional scientist, but they will convey an overall picture of drug discovery and drug action to an intelligent reader.

No attempt is made to describe various diseases and drug treatments that may help a patient's specific complaint. Those with persisting complaints are advised to see their physician.

Nearly twenty years ago, the British Nobelist Sir Peter Medawar wrote "We all nowadays give too much thought to the material blessings or evils that science has brought with it, and too little to its power to liberate us from the confinements of ignorance and superstition." This book should fulfill some of the longings for knowledge about many of the various medications that have made our lives safer, more tolerable, and happier.

Drugs, like all chemicals, react with other chemicals either in a laboratory container or in the body, whether that of an animal or a human being. The mission and fate of these chemicals in the body are emphasized because that is why we take drugs. However, some medications administered only by physicians, such as general anesthetics, have been omitted.

The section on drugs of abuse, which have given the term *drug* a bad name, treats their origin and performance the same way as sections on medicines for kidney ailments, heart failure, or asthma. However, causes of drug abuse, both biological and sociological, are also considered.

On the whole, physicians between the ages of thirty and fifty-five are the most knowledgeable about the choice and effectiveness of medications. Experience in prescribing a drug is essential in implementing a diagnosis. Such experience can be gathered by reading the current medical literature—journals and monographs—and by paying close attention to the drug inserts provided by the manufacturers of each drug. However, in order to protect himself from malpractice suits, the manufacturer usually includes every advantage and drawback in the pamphlet accompanying the drug package. That is where personal experience helps the physician in choosing a prescription. If two patients present the same complaint and the same apparent nuances of their symptoms, it will be easy to prescribe the same drug in both cases. If these nuances differ and if the life-style and the diets of the two patients are not the same, the dosage or even the specific drug may have to be altered.

Too little attention is paid in medical education to drug interactions and drug incompatibilities. Until recently the role of nutrition and diet in the control of disease has also not been taught adequately in the medical school curriculum. Younger doctors may have a better insight into these important problems.

Drugs and People

Medications, Their History and Origins, and the Way They Act

Drugs: Historical Beginnings

Drugs are chemical compounds that modify the way the body works. Most people think that these biological activities should help or heal sick people or animals. There is, however, no known drug that is not harmful or even poisonous at high doses, and much of the scientific work on drugs has attempted to widen the gap between effective and toxic doses.

The word *drug* has acquired bad connotations in recent years since the widespread abuse of a few chemicals that affect the central nervous system has become a serious sociological problem. Nevertheless, drugs act on many other organs in the body, can benefit as well as harm the nervous system, and have made possible a revolution in the way modern doctors treat disease.

Just as there is no health benefit without potential toxicity, there is no absolute goodness about drugs. However, their enormous health benefits outweigh the drawbacks in individual cases. The history, discovery, manufacture, action, acceptance, and rejection of drugs are the themes of this book.

It used to be said that what distinguishes man from animals is that people take drugs. This old adage is no longer quite true. Rats and monkeys that have been addicted experimentally to some drugs will inject themselves with those drugs to support their addiction. But otherwise the old saying still holds.

The history of drugs is shrouded in the beginning of the human race. Alcohol was made, drunk, and used to excess as far back as memory and records go. Tobacco *(Nicotiana)*, hemp *(Cannabis)*, opium poppy *(Papaver)*, and other plants containing drugs have been chewed and smoked almost as long, and coffee has been served in the Mideast throughout that area's history.

Apes and humans are believed to have taken their separate evolutionary ways some five to ten million years ago. In those times, prehumans, almost humans, and later nomadic groups of obviously human individuals roamed the landscape in search of food and shelter. The driving forces behind this foraging behavior were the need to defend themselves against the environment and to reproduce their species. The earliest humans were often threatened by malnutrition or even starvation; by predators—both animal and competing or cannibalistic human hunters; by climatic changes; and last but not least, by parasites and degenerative diseases. The kindling and taming of fire was one of a few positive contributions that further separated humans from animals. Fire gave primitive nomads some protection from cold and a way to make food more palatable.

The earliest records of their short and deprived years, estimated as no more than a couple of decades, are wall paintings and carvings on rocks that have endured for thousands of years in jungles or deserts. The pictures give us little insight into any healing arts those forebears may have invented. Probably accidental discovery of the healing powers of roots, barks, leaves, and berries and of nutritional sources of proteins and starch occurred even during those earliest stages.

Only recently, ten-to-twenty thousand years ago, nomadic tribes began to settle down in some parts of the world and formed small agricultural communities. This was one of the most profound changes in the history of the human race. Planting seeds, domesticating animals, and erecting permanent shelters for man and beast improved nutrition, provided more comfortable, though still primitive, living accommodations, and started the societal bonds that developed for better or worse into villages, towns, and cities where the first truly historical times began.

At this stage, when people began to live close together, certain rules were established to bring needed order out of unstructured conglomerated living. Strong individuals emerged as the leaders of tribal or village communities. Part of their power came from the personal help they could give to sick, wounded, and otherwise afflicted members of their group. The medicine man, witch doctor, shaman, or whatever name he went by was the first person to turn to in distress. Sometimes authority lay in an influential woman who functioned as priestess, nurse, and midwife. In most cases, power, enforced by superstition, centered in a dominant male recognized as healer, priest, judge, and leader in peace and war. A knowledge of healing herbs formed part of his power base and prerogatives, while among his duties was applying such healing products when needed.

Botanical specimens taken from trees, shrubs, and other plants formed the mainstay of most of these early medicines. Sometimes the shaman deepened the mystery of the power of his medication by adding parts of animals, both warm- and cold-blooded, and even human hearts. Some mind-induced (psychosomatic) illnesses were probably improved by suggestions, just as they are today. Also, some functional disorders responded to the active chemicals in suitably chosen plants. It must have been hard for a medicine man to decide which plant to give a patient. Trial and error was the order of his day.

Even after a healing effect was found in a certain plant, it was probably used for a variety of illnesses, whether identical in symptoms or only vaguely similar. Modern physicians still face complicated choices in diagnosis and drug therapy in spite of help from analytical tests, X-rays, ultrasound, nuclear magnetic resonance visualization, blood cell counts, urinalysis, and other laboratory aids. Imagine the dilemma of an ancient medicine man who was guided only by vague symptoms such as a generalized pain, nausea, fever, or convulsions. In such a dilemma, and without any knowledge of anatomy or pathology, some herbal concoction was given in the hope that it would work. The medicine man undoubtedly added prayers or exorcisms to the medication and believed sincerely that his ministrations would aid the afflicted.

Cynical healers also appeared. In Roman times, predictions about world affairs as well as the course of a patient's disease were based on the inspection of the intestines of newly slaughtered chickens. There was a saying that described one of these healer-seers (called a haruspex) encountering another member of the guild: *haruspex, haruspicem videns ridet* ("When one haruspex sees another, he laughs").

EARLY RECORDS OF NATURAL DRUGS

Fortunately, some medicine men and women were careful observers who had a patient's recovery uppermost in mind. Especially those who had risen to power and influence and had a scientific bent or deep compassion could be relied upon to search for valid explanations of their findings. One of the oldest, if not the oldest, records of such medicinal recommendations is found in the writings of the Chinese scholar-emperor Shen Nung, who lived in 2735 B.C., or 4720 B.P. (before the present). He compiled a book about herbs, a forerunner of the medieval pharmacopoeias that listed all the then-known medications. He was able to judge the value of some Chinese herbs. For example, he found that *Ch'ang Shan* was helpful in treating "fevers." Such fevers were, and still are, caused by malaria parasites. The drug consists of the powdered roots of a plant in the breakstone family (Saxifragaceae, now identified as *Dichroa febrifuga*, Lour.) It took almost 4700 years before a group of Chinese chemists isolated two compounds (the dichroines) from the plants, one of which later proved to control bird malaria. The leaves of this plant—called *Shun Chi* or *chuine* in present-day China—also contain antimalarial chemicals (the febrifugines), one of which is identical with one of the dichroines. These alkaloids (organic bases) were studied and synthesized during World War II in an effort to protect Americans from malaria in the Pacific and other tropical campaigns. Chemists were never successful, however, because they could not separate the nausea they produced from their antimalarial effects.

The old emperor Shen Nung also observed the stimulating effect of another ancient Chinese medicinal plant, Ma Huang. This one, now called *Ephedra sinica*, contains a number of alkaloids, chief of which, ephedrine, was isolated by the Japanese chemist Nagai in 1887, over 4600 years after the effect of the plant had been recorded. Ephedrine and some closely related compounds are responsible for the ability of the wiry plant to stimulate blood pressure and breathing. The drug also contracts blood vessels.

The 5000-year tradition of natural drugs continues to flourish in China even today. A philosophy curious to us underlies their reasoning. Diseases are evil occurrences that are counteracted by good influences, they say, and Nature is good and therefore healing. The traditional Chinese physicians overlook the fact that Nature is not always kind. Apart from cataclysms like earthquakes and hurricanes that threaten all life, many parts of medicinal plants are toxic, often deadly poisonous. The history both of intentional assassinations and suicides and of accidental poisoning by swallowing certain plant products, as well as the killing of game and enemies with curare-tipped arrows, are witness to the widespread toxicity of botanical materials. Some Chinese pharmacognosists have claimed that synthetic compounds with no structural resemblance to harmless natural products are more dangerous than naturally occurring plant constituents, but this claim is unsubstantiated. Some synthetic compounds are highly toxic, others are not, and the same is true of natural products. In thousands of cases, chemical manipulation of their structure has lessened the toxicity of natural alkaloids, antibiotics, hormones, snake venoms, and other biologically active substances. Frequently these semisynthetic chemical cousins or analogs can be used in clinical medicine much more safely than their natural ancestors.

Much knowledge of early drugs has been lost from every civilization. What remains is passed on in sporadically recorded epics and folklore unearthed by archeologists and linguistic scholars. Tropical and subtropical regions, with their greater variety of plants, have given us most of the descriptions of these medicines. Although some ancient drugs have survived throughout the ages and in a refined form are still used, they amount to a small percentage of modern medications.

Ancient Hindu records mention eating chaulmoogra fruit to treat leprosy. We now know that it contains several oils not very effective against leprosy bacteria. Treating the disfigured areas with these oils has been replaced entirely by swallowing dapsone, a synthetic drug, or by other medicines.

A treatment still in use in underdeveloped regions for some intestinal problems is ipecac, the powdered roots of ipecacuanha *(Cephaelis ipecacuanha* or *C. acuminata)*. These plants were already being used by Brazilian Indians before the European conquest; they treated "bloody flux," a form of amebic diarrhea, with "igpecaya." Samuel Purchas in *Purchas his Pilgrims* published a description of this material in 1615. As often happens in medicine, the successful recovery of a highly placed person made treatment with a new drug popular. In the case of ipecacuanha, the dauphin, son of Louis XIV, was cured of his amebic infection by the physician Helvetius towards the end of the seventeenth century. Yet amebiasis was not studied intensively until 1875, and another thirty-five years passed before extraction of ipecac showed that the alkaloids emetine and cephaline were the active ingredients of the plant. Ipecac had been used for centuries to make poisoned people vomit; unfortunately, this property has limited the use of emetine for curing amebiasis.

Mediterranean peoples formerly pulverized the dried flower heads of species in the ragweed family, especially *Artemesia maritima*, to get rid of intestinal worms. This plant is native to south-central Russia. Its active ingredient, santonin, was synthesized by British and Swiss organic chemists, yet all the studies have not been able to separate clinically effective doses from toxic ones. However, santonin is still used for roundworm infections in farm animals.

Another plant used to treat worms is goose-foot *(Chenopodium anthelminticum)*. From its flowers comes a volatile oil that contains the active principle, ascaridole. The Romans gave it the name Chenopodium; the Hebrews called it Jerusalem Oak; and others dub it Mexican tea.

Likewise, a dark-green, thick oil can be pressed from the male fern *(Dryopteris filix mas)* that helps to expel tapeworms. This plant's use is ancient. Its active ingredient is also ascaridole. In humans it is effective only at almost toxic doses, and it is prescribed mostly in veterinary medicine. Its use by early medicine men emphasizes their need of medications regardless of side effects. Many of these antique natural drugs would be unacceptable to today's regulatory agencies such as the Food and Drug Administration, as well as to the medical profession.

South and Central American Indians made many prehistoric discoveries of drug-bearing plants. Mexican Aztecs even recorded their properties in hieroglyphics on rocks, but our knowledge of their studies comes mainly from manuscripts of Spanish monks and medical men attached to the forces of the conquistador Cortez.

Pre-Columbian Mexicans used many things, from tobacco *(Nicotiana)* to mind-expanding (hallucinogenic) plants, in their medicinal collections. The most fascinating of these are sacred mushrooms, used in religious ceremonies to induce altered states of the mind, not just drunkenness. In the recent past, many of these mushrooms as well as flowers and shrubs have been extracted chemically and their active ingredients identified. For example, peyote, a small cactus, now named *Lophophora williamsii*, contains alkaloids, especially mescaline, that cause hallucinations. The Indians called sacred mushrooms *teonacatl* (Nahuatl: "God's flesh"). Some of these belong to *Psilobe* species and contain hallucinogens (psilocine, psilocybine). These and other plants that produced temporary insane (psychotic) reactions were abhorred by the Spanish priests, who saw their use as rites of the devil.

Other South American Indians, especially those in the Peruvian Andes mountains, made several early discoveries of drug-bearing plants. Two of these contain alkaloids of worldwide importance that have become permanent drugs. They are cocaine and quinine.

COCAINE

Cocaine is extracted from leaves, especially from *Erythroxylon coca*, a bushy shrub native in South American countries at high altitudes, such as Bolivia, Peru, Ecuador, and Chile. Cocaine is the primary alkaloid in these leaves. Its numbing effect was long known, although its clinical use as a local anesthetic had to await the studies of the Austrian physician Carl Köller about one hundred years ago. Another property of cocaine is mental stimulation, which can lead to addiction. This potential for addiction that physicians call dependence liability, as well as the stimulation, was known and used with sinister intent by Indian chiefs hundreds of years ago. The chiefs maintained a messenger system along the spine of the Andes in order to control their thinly populated kingdoms, stretched for thousands of miles along the mountains and isolated from each other by the rugged terrain. The messengers had to run at high altitudes and needed stimulants for this exhausting task. Their princely employers provided the runners with coca leaves for this purpose and enslaved them further by paying them with more coca leaves, thus maintaining the addiction for which the poor runners were willing to continue their never-ending jobs. When coca leaves reached Europe with the Spanish conquistadores, they led to one of the first waves of euphoric hallucinogenic drugs.

QUININE

Quinine was isolated from the bark of the cinchona tree by Caventou and Pelletier in 1820, two hundred years after the bark was introduced into Europe for the treatment of malaria. The Peruvian Indians had recognized for years the value of the quinquina tree for treating feverish patients. Some historians believe that malaria was imported to South America by the conquistadores and their African slaves. A persistent story exists about Dona Francisca Henriquez de Ribera, wife of Count Chinchon, the Spanish viceroy of Peru. She fell ill with malaria (the "tertians" variety with chills and fever that recur every third day) and was cured by an Indian healer who gave her the bark. In gratitude for the cure, the countess distributed the bark to other patients in Lima and thus alerted Spanish physicians to its clinical potential. The great Swedish botanist Linnaeus (Karl von Linné, 1707–78) later called the tree cinchona in honor of Countess Chinchon, mispelling her name in the process. It is improbable that the countess persuaded Spanish doctors to use the bark, because she died in Cartagena, Columbia, in 1641, while returning home. As the antimalarial value of cinchona became more widely recognized while supplies of the bark fell short of demand, the cost of the powder was often matched by its weight in gold.

The cinchona tree grows wild in the sub-Andean jungles, and a number of European powers tried to transplant it to other tropical places. Peruvian officials realized what a gold mine these trees represented and strictly prohibited their export. A British attempt to smuggle some trees out of Peru failed, but two Dutch adventurers managed to get a few specimens across the border. The stolen trees were taken to Java and became the ancestors of later improved plantation trees that, before 1940, furnished 97 percent of the world's supply of quinine.

The inaccessibility of Java—and of Sri Lanka, where a few smaller plantations existed—became a source of worry for European drug factories that were the principal sources of pure quinine. This concern was felt acutely by German manufacturers in World War I, when they were unable to supply European colonies in Africa with the drug. In World War II, British and American suppliers also were cut off from their oriental sources of quinine when the Japanese occupied Java and Malay. In both instances, the drug shortage stimulated intensive research to surmount this handicap, and the resulting new compounds are almost the only effective synthetic antimalarials we have today. Nevertheless, quinine has kept a modest but important and inexpensive place in antimalarial treatment.

HISTORY OF INORGANIC DRUGS

As the centuries unrolled and new civilizations appeared, cultural, artistic, and medical developments shifted toward the new centers of power. A reversal of the traditional search for botanical drugs occurred in Greece in the fourth century B.C. (about 2500 B.P.), when Hippocrates (estimated dates, 460–377 B.C.), the "Father of Medicine," became interested in inorganic salts as medications.

Hippocrates' authority lasted throughout the Middle Ages and reminded alchemists and medical experimenters of the potential of inorganic drugs. In fact, a distant descendant of Hippocrates' prescriptions was the use of antimony salts in elixirs (alcoholic solutions) advocated by Basilius Valentius in the middle of the fifteenth century, and by the medical alchemist Philipus Aureolus Paracelsus (born Theophrastus Bombastus von Hohenheim, in Switzerland, 1493–1541). The ethics of Hippocrates as incorporated in the physicians' Hippocratic oath have survived better than his preference for inorganic salts.

However, we still use magnesium sulfate (named Epsom salt for the British town of Epsom), both internally and externally; aluminum salt astringents; sodium and potassium chlorides and calcium salts for various deficiencies; barium sulfate as an X ray contrast agent; and sodium iodide to prevent thyroid disorders, as well as stannous fluoride to prevent tooth decay. Gold compounds are just now experiencing a renaissance in the treatment of arthritis, and silver nitrate had been used to protect the eyes of newborn infants from gonorrheal blindness before penicillin took its place. Lithium salts are used in gout and to smooth out the biphasic phase of manic-depression. Many heavy metals are incorporated as traces in diet supplements, since they have been recognized as essential parts of important biological catalysts.

The next great—and reactionary—influence on medicinal thought came from the Greek physician from Pergamum, Claudius Galenus, or Galen (131–200 A.D.), who taught in Rome. Galenic medicine consisted of preparations of plants by soaking (infusion) or boiling (decoction). As Oliver Wendell Holmes said, "These Galenists were what we should call herb doctors today." Galen claimed that herbal mixtures could provide all the essentials for health and therefore could be applied to all conceivable health defects. He was an early vegetarian.

We know today that a strict vegetarian diet, without milk, cheese, eggs, etc., cannot contain all the protein-building amino acids needed for normal growth and body maintenance. In Galen's storeroom *(apotheke)* some metallic substances such as copper and zinc ores, iron sulfate, and cadmium oxide were still present, probably as a tribute to Hippocrates' drug inventory. Galen insisted on carefully identifying the kind and age of botanical materials and thus foreshadowed the value of controlling the purity of drugs. Among his favorite and potent drugs were hyoscyamus (which contains atropine), opium (the source of morphine), and squill (which contains heart stimulants, cardiac glycosides similar to digitalis).

SOME MEDIEVAL MEDICINES

Galen's teachings made such a profound impact on medieval society and medicine that they were followed for over a thousand years. In western Europe, where medical knowledge was encased in Catholic monasteries, Galen's prescriptions were embraced and almost embalmed by the conservative monks. Although some teachings of contemporary Islamic scholars filtered into this environment, many centuries had to pass before herbal medicine could be replaced by newer treatments.

After the fall of the Roman and Byzantian empires and the rise of Islam in the Middle East, "the civilized world" of Europe was in decline. The migration of Eastern peoples, the constant and cruel wars all over the continent, and the absence of cultural and intellectual life-styles made scholarly studies of drugs impossible. The herb gardens of monasteries were the chief source of healing plants, but infections, heart disease, cancer ("a fire in her bowels"), and the innumerable battle wounds and disfigurements from torture could not be treated rationally. Plagues swept across the Continent and the British Isles, chiefly bubonic plague, viral pandemics, and later syphilis. The victims were layed to rest in mass graves with no medicines to ease their final agonies. Life was hard and, on the average, short; at fifty or fifty-five a person was very old, over the hill, an ancient senior citizen; most died in their forties or sooner.

Bleeding the patient by opening a vein or with leeches was one of the few medical treatments and was used for various ills; amputations of wounded or badly infected limbs was carried out without anesthesia or benefit of soap-and-water hygiene; cesarean deliveries meant the cruel and certain death of the mother.

These desperate health conditions applied to kings and serfs alike for almost fifteen hundred years. No wonder that a better life could be imagined only in the heavens, a hypothesis that has never been proved.

The little that was known about healing plants, minerals and tissues was called materia medica, a term still used for drug information at the turn of this century. Latin was used throughout the collective accounts of this subject because that was the professional language of the monks and also because it kept the common people in ignorance. We would not condone this procedure today, yet we know that many patients do suffer from mentally triggered physical symptoms after hearing a diagnosis of their conditions.

When pamphlets could no longer hold the accumulating knowledge of materia medica, larger, more formal collections were gathered in national pharmacopoeias. The first of these books appeared in Florence (1498, six years after Columbus landed in Haiti), followed by others in Nuremberg (1535), Basel (1561), Augsburg 1564), and London (1618). Standards of purity and methods of preparing various drug products accompanied the descriptions of botanical and mineralogical specimens. One amusing item tells how to make a sort of candy of red rose petals for pale tired people and of white roses for those with too ruddy complexions.

The late middle ages coincided with the upsurge of alchemy, a primitive chemistry dealing mostly with inorganic substances. The renewed interest in inorganic materials pushed botanical sources of medicines into second place temporarily. True, quinine (cinchona) appeared during that century, but the next great botanical drug, digitalis, was not introduced until the end of the 1700s.

2

Discovery of Early Modern Medicines

DIGITALIS

In 1785 the British physician William Withering published a book entitled *An Account of the Foxglove and Some of its Medical Uses: with Practical Remarks on Dropsy and Other Diseases*. Dropsy, characterized by the accumulation of fluid (edema) as with congestive heart failure, had previously been treated with dried and powdered purple foxglove *(Digitalis purpurea)*, which is still grown as an ornamental flower. But digitalis had remained a typical Galenic drug used also for skin ulcers, epilepsy, and other poorly diagnosed diseases. Withering himself had no clear picture of the cause of edema but noticed in passing that digitalis powerfully affected the heart. It took another fourteen years for John Ferriar (1799) to sort out the ability of digitalis to increase the contraction of heart muscles and to understand that its diuretic effect on the kidney, which increases the secretion and flow of urine, was secondary to this action.

The compounds responsible for the action of digitalis have complicated chemical structures called cardiac glycosides, and occur in a number of plants. Similarly, squill, the dried, fleshy bulb of the sea onion *(Urginea maritima)* had been used medicinally in ancient Egypt, and the Romans also used it as a heart tonic and kidney stimulant. In stronger, more toxic doses, this material was used to cause vomiting and even as a rat poison.

The seeds of *Strophanthus* also contain cardiac glycosides and were used in African arrow poisons. Other sources of these heart stimulants are skins of common toads, which figured in ancient Chinese folk medicine and in European medieval prescriptions until replaced by digitalis. The purple foxglove had been known botanically since 1250, when it was mentioned by Welch physicians, but it was named in 1542 by the botanist Fuchsius.

The individual digitalis glycosides are hard to separate, but a few have been purified. Fairly well purified preparations are available commercially, but because they cannot be reliably analyzed chemically, they must be evaluated biologically. For example, their effect on heart contraction is measured on the toad heart. A purified glycoside from another kind of digitalis *(D. lanata)*, called digoxin and taken orally, is probably the most widely prescribed and satisfactory digitalis product in modern heart treatment.

Although the isolation of pure cardiac glycosides had to await the development of modern ways to separate closely related chemicals, the introduction of digitalis was one of the earliest steps in modern drug therapy. During the period following the American, the French, and the beginning of the Industrial Revolutions, shackles of medieval thought patterns were shed and explanations of drug actions were sought. Several botanical drugs were therefore extracted, purified, and concentrated. Then the residue was chemically fractioned in order to isolate individual components of the usually gummy mixtures.

OPIATES

The first example of a natural product that fits into this account historically is opium and its alkaloids. Alkaloids are natural substances that are chemically alkaline or basic. Opium is obtained by cutting surfaces of unripe seed capsules of the oriental poppy *(Papaver somniferum)*, which spread from Asia Minor to many Mediterranean and Southeast Asian countries. It is also grown in American gardens for its brilliant flowers. A milky juice oozes from the wounded seed box and is dried in the air. The brown gummy residue is powdered. The word *opium* is derived from a Greek word meaning "juice." Even before the ancient Greeks encountered it, the Sumerians (Babylonians) carved tablets with pictures of the poppy about 6000

B.P., along with the inscription *hul* ("joy") and *gil* ("plant"), and apparently were aware of the mind-affecting effects of opium.

The Greek naturalist Theophrastus (died about 287 B.C.) mentioned poppy juice in his writing. During the rise of Arabian-Islamic medicine, opium was used widely and introduced to Oriental peoples, principally as a constipant to control dysentery (our paregoric). With Islamic inroads into Europe during the sixteenth century, opium was introduced there and became widely accepted. Paracelsus (1493–1544) made a purified preparation of poppy juice that he called laudanum, which can still be purchased in some drug stores today.

About twenty-five opium alkaloids are responsible for the drug actions of opium. The main one is morphine. It is a powerful analgesic (painkiller); in fact, it serves as a standard for all other natural and synthetic analgesics. Morphine also constipates by slowing down peristalsis, the involuntary muscle contractions that move the contents of the intestines on their course. It also depresses respiration, causes sleepiness, and has several other minor activities. Mentally, morphine produces euphoria, a sensation of well-being, and after repeated use, dependence liability (addiction).

A minor alkaloid of opium is codeine, which depresses the cough reflex much better than morphine. Codeine is still used in cough medicines, although it is usually displaced by synthetic compounds with fewer side effects. Codeine is an effective constipant but only a fairly good analgesic agent. It is slightly addictive.

Papaverine, another minor opium alkaloid, does not relieve pain, but because it dilates arteries well, it has some value in painful angina pectoris. Like codeine, papaverine is manufactured synthetically. Noscapine (narcotine) is a minor opium derivative that is beginning to enjoy acceptance as a cough medicine (antitussive). None of the other opium alkaloids are used as drugs, and many of them are toxic. Obviously, the various alkaloids in opium possess complex and often contradictory activities.

Some derivatives of morphine are stronger pain relievers than morphine itself: for example, the synthetic drug heroin. Unfortunately, heroin also is more addictive than morphine and has become the most dreaded and abused pleasure-producing (euphoriant) drug. Smoking opium in specially constructed pipes has been practiced for centuries in Oriental opium dens and even in French literary salons. A major wave of abuse of opium and its relatives has flooded the world in the twentieth century and shows no signs of receding. However, other chemicals such as cocaine and some synthetics with more psychosis-producing (psychotomimetic) properties have displaced opiates in some parts of the world.

ANTICHOLINERGICS

Belladonna drugs, which have been studied for over 150 years, also come from alkaloid-bearing plants. The name *Atropa belladonna* was coined by Linné in the eighteenth century for the deadly nightshade vine to remind us of the poisonous nature of this plant known to writers of the Hindu Veda and to other authors in Roman and medieval times. Atropos was one of the Greek "Fates" who cut the thread of life. Large doses of extracts from belladonna were used to cause insidious and hard-to-trace deaths from its poison. Because weak extracts also dilate the pupil of the eye, renaissance women used belladonna to make their eyes appear more brilliant, hence the name *bella donna* ("beautiful lady").

The alkaloid atropine was isolated in 1831 but later recognized as a mixture of chemicals with mirror-opposite structures called optical antipodes (the hyoscyamines, named after the henbane shrub, *Hyoscyamus niger*). Atropine also occurs in *Datura stramonium*—called variously thornapple, stinkweed, and jimson weed (because it was found near Jamestown, Virginia). Another important alkaloid, scopolamine, was named after the plant *Scopolia carniolica*, but it also occurs together with atropine in henbane.

Atropine is used widely in medicine. In small, nontoxic doses it slows down secretion by glands and therefore helps in drying up unwanted fluids during operations. Dentists use it to control saliva. Atropine also acts as a powerful antispasmodic drug to prevent spastic contractions of involuntary muscles such as those of the gullet, stomach, and intestines, over which people have no conscious control. This antispasmodic activity extends to muscles in the eye, and therefore atropine has been used in the past to dilate the pupils in order to see inside the eye.

Scopolamine has similar properties, but these are overshadowed by its effects on the brain. In suitable concentration this drug depresses the central nervous system causing twilight sleep, a state useful in obstetrics and minor surgical procedures. In smaller doses, injections of scopolamine used as a truth serum in interrogations produce the relaxation necessary to gain the subject's cooperation.

Both atropine and scopolamine work by counteracting the neurohormone acetylcholine, which will be discussed later and which does many different things. Drugs with many different actions are not as valuable as those that do one or two things, and therefore thousands of attempts have been made to develop chemical relatives (synthetic analogs) of atropine and scopolamine that have fewer actions. Because these alkaloids have a reasonably simple ester-type of structure, chemists have altered one section of their molecules after another in these attempts. However, none of the antispasmodics found have proved appreciably better than the natural ones. Somewhat more specific drugs have been developed as dilators of the eye (mydriatics) such as homatropine, but a substance that only relaxes the intestinal tract, which would be of particular use for intestinal ulcers, has not been found. The main advantage of some of these synthetic and less powerful antispasmodics is their decreased depression of the central nervous system.

Development, Naming, and Introduction of Medicinal Agents

No drug has just one effect. The medically desirable actions are invariably accompanied by side effects. Such near-toxic or clearly poisonous results must be balanced against the clinical advantages of the substance. Much of this becomes apparent in animal experiments, although the final value of a drug is determined through clinical trials and broad experience with patients.

The progress of almost all new drugs is quite similar. The drug is announced with fanfare in medical journals, at scientific meetings, and by the news media. Although hedged today in increasingly cautious language, claims of the drug's performance are usually encouraging. Within a year or two, wide use of the substance by millions of patients will inevitably disclose unwanted side effects, some serious, and both physicians and patients often become cautious of its use. Generally, the percentage of side effects is relatively small, and when put into proper perspective, the ratio of benefit to risk becomes more acceptable. Then the drug wins a more permanent niche in the arsenal of medicinal agents.

In many parts of the world, drugs are dispensed in apothecary stores with a counter behind which a druggist works. They sell chiefly medical supplies. Their licensed pharmacists used to spend the greater part of their time compounding drugs and additives as prescribed by physicians. In this country such stores are called drugstores but are really department stores, the successors to the general stores of old. Nowadays pharmacists buy drugs in ready-to-take forms from wholesale distributors or directly from pharmaceutical manufacturers whose sales personnel (detail men and women) visit the drugstores and take their orders. The same detail people also visit physicians and leave samples and descriptive pamphlets about their company's drugs. Like ready-to-eat foods, most drugs have been standardized in this manner, and the labor of measuring and mixing is done by machines in the manufacturers' plants.

In the West, this standardization has existed for a long time. In the East, natural drugs are still largely preferred to synthetics. Perhaps tradition and a deference to the economics of horticulture play roles in this attitude. There have been similar cases of agricultural concern in Europe and America. One of them followed the introduction of synthetic indigo, a blue dye originally obtained by fermenting *Indigofera tinctoria*. This plant had been grown in highly profitable plantations in South Carolina that were ruined by the appearance of the purer tint of the cheaper synthetic indigo. Fortunately, other economic specialty crops soon took the place of the plant.

Tobacco planters belong in this category. Tobacco is a very profitable crop and the basis of a vast agricultural and industrial enterprise. Several areas in the United States, Asia Minor, and Africa derive their principal revenues from tobacco *(Nicotiana tabaccum)*. Next to grain alcohol, tobacco is probably the most widely used and abused crude drug in the world, yet many of its constituents, especially the nicotiana alkaloids and tobacco smoke have a variety of toxic effects. The two-phase action of nicotine and the minor tobacco alkaloids consists of briefly stimulating and then depressing certain centers (ganglia) in the cerebral cortex of the brain. This leads to an overall calming not unlike that produced by tranquilizers, a pleasant feeling desired by a large percentage of the world's population. Therefore physical dependence on tobacco is almost as hard to shed as dependence on and tolerance of alcohol, and the raw materials for both appear destined to be grown for profit interminably.

NAMING DRUGS

The unfamiliarity of drug names is a problem for many both to pronounce and to remember. Like the drugs themselves, their names have a history. The inorganic salts were named for the elements that form them; table salt, being composed of sodium and chlorine, is called sodium chloride. However, organic chemicals are named according to strict rules that have evolved over the last 150 years. In the beginning, medicines were called according to the use of their source. For example atropine was named for its parent plant, *Atropa belladonna*; papaverine for the poppy, *Papaver somniferum*; Adrenaline for the adrenal gland; and so on. An early antifever (antipyretic) drug was called Antifebrin; an antiseptic for the urinary tract, Urotropine. These names were coined by commercial manufacturers of the drugs and bore no relation to their chemistry.

Chemical names of organic molecules can be very cumbersome. For example, the correct name of the simple structure of the antihistamine diphenhydramine, or Benadryl, is 2-diphenylmethoxy-1-N,N-dimethylaminoethane hydrochloride. Such names are systematized and brought up-to-date in *Chemical Abstracts*, a journal published by the American Chemical Society in Columbus, Ohio, and used worldwide. Who but a trained organic chemist could remember, pronounce, and decipher such chemical names?—certainly not even pharmacists who dispense drugs or physicians who prescribe and biologists who study drugs, but have forgotten the short course in organic chemistry that they took in their sophomore year in college. For this reason, a new compound while under biological study is usually given a number and the initials of the chemist who prepared it or of the company where it was made. Thus, a compound might bear such code numbers as SKF 385 (for Smith Kline & French), Win 8620 (for Sterling-Winthrop), etc.

By the time a promising compound becomes a candidate for clinical trials, it often receives a name that is easier to use. Such names have to be approved by the Council on Pharmacy and Chemistry of the American Medical Association; a few of them may in time become nonproprietary or generic names for the compounds. (See Appendix A.) Most other developed nations approve similar generic names, and the World Health Organization in Geneva, Switzerland, publishes international nonproprietary names for drugs. The American Medical Association's Council adopts the generic name (U.S. Adopted Name; USAN), then publishes it in the journal *New and*

Nonofficial Remedies. These nonproprietary names may be used by any manufacturer who has the right to market the product; they must appear on the package insert (the paper always tucked in the box with a drug), together with the dosage directions and other vital information, especially precautions and warnings of side effects. The public would do well to read these inserts.

The preferred way of forming the name of a drug is by a pleasant sounding contraction of its chemical name. For example, the generic name of tranylcypromine (a drug to help depression, and synthesized at the University of Virginia) is derived from its chemical name, *tran*s-2-phen*ylcyclo**pro*pyl*amine*. The trademarked name of this drug is Parnate. The *-ate* ending comes from sulfate, the commercially marketed salt of the compound. Since the acid or the basic ion that forms the salt of an acid or a basic drug, respectively, is irrelevant for the action of the compound, it is often dropped by the wayside. The local anesthetic procaine is marketed as its hydrochloride salt, but this fact is seldom mentioned; the protected trade name of the drug is Novocain, but almost no physician or dentist will tell you that they will numb your tissues with Novocain hydrochloride.

Today in the United States, all rights to market a new drug may be protected for twenty-two years following the issue of a patent. During this period, only the originating firm or inventor has exclusive rights to produce the drug. Quite commonly the manufacturer guards his interest further by registering his proprietary name as a protected trademark. Such "trade" names may not be used by any other firm or person in marketing a drug even after the patent has expired. They are capitalized and followed by the symbol ®. Trade names are chosen to be pleasant sounding, easy to remember, and easy to pronounce.

Pharmaceutical manufacturers bombard physicians with advertisements, pamphlets, and especially visits from their sales forces, who praise the advantages and uses of their proprietary drugs. Physicians, hard-pressed for time, frequently learn many of the essential facts about new drugs from these "detail" men and women, who naturally use the registered trade names in their descriptions. Usually the physician learns and remembers the trademarked word and hardly ever knows the more complicated generic name. It is safe to say that at least 90 percent of all prescriptions are written with proprietary names.

The proprietary names so widely used should be capitalized. But after several decades the original source of a drug sometimes becomes hazy and may be—unofficially—forgotten. Thus, Aspirin, Adrenalin, Novocain, Xylocaine, Atebrine, and other classical drug names were, and still are, proprietary trade names, but are seldom capitalized in the current literature and in newspapers.

After a patent has expired, any manufacturer may develop and market the drug, provided he uses the less familiar generic name, and so long as he does not infringe on protected dosage forms, shapes, and colors. In almost all cases, a generic drug is equivalent to the proprietary material. Chemically the two substances are identical because the Food and Drug Administration can make its own analytical tests and will reject any inferior product. But judging the availability of the drug in the body is harder. A chemical is usually encased in a capsule or pressed in a tablet, often with inert diluting fillers, and therefore may dissolve at a different rate in body liquids than the original proprietary product. This potential defect, although rare, could affect the availability of the drug to body tissues. Again, our regulatory governmental agencies are charged with keeping a wary eye on this possibility by measuring the speed of solution and the effects of supposedly "inert" additives.

Physicians can consult the annual editions of the *Physicians Desk Reference* for up-to-date drug names and other pertinent information. Names are listed in both generic and proprietary indices; often a drug developed simultaneously by different firms in different parts of the world may have different names. A more unified naming system (nomenclature) is therefore badly needed.

The member countries of the World Health Organization have been asked to observe the following recommendations. As with other recommendations, they are not always heeded, but they are an attempt at international unification.

1. Names should preferably be free from any anatomical, physiological, pathological, or therapeutic suggestion.

2. Names should be formed by combining syllables from the chemical name of the compound in such a way that its important chemical groups are indicated.

3. Names should not, in general, exceed four syllables, should be distinctive in sound and spelling, and should not be easily confused with names already in use. They should not end with a capital letter or a number.

HOW SCIENCE PROGRESSES

Progress in science seldom occurs in totally unexpected giant steps. Rather, one small step forward will be discovered here, another one there. Once in a while an innovative young scientist will put those scattered findings together, see how they fit, and from them make new predictions. In the case of biologically active chemicals, the age-old question of how they really work has not yet been answered, but many medicinal scientists have offered opinions, based on more or less good, experimental evidence. Take the case of time-honored aspirin. The chemical name of aspirin, acetylsalicylic acid, comes from the Latin botanical name for the willow *(Salix alba)*. For hundreds of years a sort of willow tea relieved aches and pains. But it took 71 more years from the introduction of aspirin as a drug in 1899 to the first inkling of an explanation in 1970 of how its antiinflammatory action worked. Indeed, this information had to wait for a totally unrelated event, namely, the discovery of the way in which cells biosynthesize an inflammatory, hormonelike chemical, one of the prostaglandins. This is a good example of the truth that some apparently abstract biochemical research may pay off in practical results.

If you go hunting with a gun or a bow and arrow, you aim at a target and try to hit it. Until just a few years ago and only in a very few cases since then, could anybody recognize the target of a drug, and the aim therefore remained uncertain. There had to be a target and it had to be a chemical. All drugs are chemicals, and all they can do is to react with another chemical in the cells of an animal or person. The drug has to be received by such a cell chemical, and therefore that location is called a receptor.

At the turn of the century, when this term surfaced, chemistry was not far enough advanced to suggest what a receptor might look like. The earliest attempts to make such a suggestion came from Paul Ehrlich (1854–1915), generally regarded as the father of medicinal science. Others have achieved more accurate and more specific theories and results, but they were not confronted with the void of knowledge that confronted him, and had more to build on. Ehrlich started with virtually nothing; his fine mind could compare few precedents, and yet from such bare ground, it developed an edifice of medicinal science that has survived three quarters of a century of feverish change.

Ehrlich was originally an immunologist, interested in sera and vaccines. In a way this was prophetic, since we believe now, one hundred years later, that the portions of nucleic acids called genes program the formation of perhaps a hundred thousand or more antibodies that help "normal" individuals to withstand the unending attacks of environmental, nutritional, and infectious substances foreign to the body. Ehrlich thought that receptors are protrusions of cell membranes. Even though we know now that such a picture is naive, echoes of these ideas still abound. Many antibodies are located on cell membranes, and their often huge protein molecules project true acidic, basic, and neutral side chains from the continuous protein (peptide) backbone. Drugs, according to Ehrlich, are attracted to receptors by side chains called haptophores (from the Greek meaning "to bear a fastening"). In modern terms these could be equated with the weak molecular attractions exerted by large protein molecules or nucleic acids. The points of bonding between drug and receptor would correspond, in present concepts, to the "active sites" of enzymes and similar large biological catalysts. We also believe now that there may be more than one active site on an enzyme molecule, and that occupation of site number 2 can deform the shape of the enzyme and thereby ruin accessibility to active site number 1, which is needed for normal functioning. Ehrlich had similar ideas in mind when he explained toxic side effects of drugs by the occupation of toxicophoric side chains. He thus approached the theoretical foundation for the understanding of the action of at least some drugs and anticipated the modern development of molecular pharmacology.

Equally impressive were Ehrlich's arrangements in practical matters. He taught us that we should study contemporary problems in human and animal health. It may be harder to work on such topics, but the intellectual and public rewards of such studies are worth the extra effort. In his day, venereal diseases menaced large sections of the population. Ehrlich attacked these problems by systematically synthesizing over 1,000 organic compounds designed to kill spirochetes, the microbes causing syphilis. He also made hundreds of compounds for tests against trypanosomes that cause human sleeping sickness in tropical regions and similar diseases of horses and cattle in Africa. Unfortunately, the hope that this research would contribute to healthy living and to agriculture in the then colonial countries in East Africa was not realized.

At that time radioactive tracers, now so common in biological experiments, were undreamed of. However, microbes had to be seen in order for their life processes to be followed with some certainty. A number of early microbiologists succeeded in selectively staining microbes without equally staining surrounding tissues. The most durable of these staining methods was worked out by Christoph Gram (1884). Ehrlich and others used dyes to visualize microbes under the microscope. It occurred to him that if such dyes were synthetically linked with toxic atoms or groups of atoms, they might kill dangerous microbes with a minimum damage to the tissues of the host. This concept became the basis of chemotherapy, a term Ehrlich coined in 1891. Even though using the selective toxicity of dyestuffs in therapy is largely a thing of the past, drug selectivity has remained the prime goal of all medicinal science.

WHO MAKES DRUGS TODAY AND HOW THEY GO ABOUT IT

The second problem Ehrlich attacked—and solved—was how to develop a useful medicine in the most successful way. The first concept of a new drug always arises in the mind of one clever inventor. But from there on, many minds and hands will become involved. The compound must be synthesized or isolated by chemists in sufficient quantity and as inexpensively as possible. Relations of chemical structure to biological activity must be explored by making chemical analogs, often hundreds of them, in order to identify the most powerful, least toxic, and most suitable member of a series of related chemicals. The chemists work in close cooperation with pharmacologists and microbiologists, who have to develop fast, practical, and valid tests for screening all those compounds. This kind of cooperation is hard to get in universities. Intellectual freedom as it is found in academic research departments often lures scientists into personal side roads. Chemists may want to study a variety of interesting reactions of their compounds; the biologists, located in other parts of town or even in other cities, may undertake the study of cellular and microbial matters unrelated to the development of the drug. These excursions delay and sidetrack the main objective of the cooperative work areas although they might lead to valuable insights in other fields.

The only two types of institutions where close cooperation takes place between scientists in different areas of medicinal research are private and governmental research institutes and the laboratories of the pharmaceutical industry. Ehrlich solicited private foundations to support his work and founded a research institute in which organic chemists, toxicologists, microbiologists, pharmacologists, biochemists, parasitologists, and physicians surrounded him. In such close quarters ideas are constantly exchanged, with the result that chemists become at least token biologists; physicians grope for the underlying principles of their art; and experimental biologists begin to think in biochemical terms. Yet an atmosphere of academic freedom in such institutes will allow and even encourage the scientists to explore questions that might have a bearing on their common goal.

Institutes of this type have sprung up in many parts of the world, wherever the wealth of private individuals, foundations or governmental support has made them possible. The Pasteur Institutes in Paris and other locations, the Salk Institute in La Jolla, California, the National Institutes of Health outside of Washington, D.C., and the Central Drug Research Institute in Lucknow, India, are some examples. Laboratories with a more narrowly defined goal but equally high scientific standards are the Sloan-Kettering Institute for Cancer Research in New York, the Southern Research Institute in Birmingham, Alabama, the Center of Cancer Research in Fox Chase, Pennsylvania, the Institutes for Tropical Diseases and Cancer in London, some of the German Max Planck Institutes, and the Istituto Superiore de Sanità in Rome. Some of these have links with large hospitals, but not at the expense of their research. Rather, they have become a breeding ground for outstanding medical discoveries and have harbored several Nobel Prize winners.

Intermediate between these institutes and the strictly goal-oriented pharmaceutical industry are such laboratories as those of the Wellcome Foundation and the Roche Foundation, both of which are financed by their parent industries, the Burroughs-Wellcome Corporation and Hoffmann-LaRoche Inc., respectively. These companies plough back some of their profits into biomedical research with barely any strings attached. The resulting findings go not only to the parent companies but also freely into the open literature. These industrial foundations also have attracted prominent biomedical scientists.

The chief sources of new drugs have been, and are, the laboratories of the research-minded pharmaceutical industry. Of the hundreds listed as pharmaceutical firms, not more than forty all over the world possess facilities that produce the increasingly complex drugs that have transformed modern medicine. They are located primarily in Belgium, Britain, France, Germany, Italy, Japan, Scandinavia,

Switzerland, and the United States. Many of them are multinational corporations with production and sales organizations in many parts of the world, but their research to discover and develop new drugs is usually done at their home base unless tax, import, and monopoly laws favor a dispersion or even a duplication of effort in other countries.

WHY DRUGS ARE EXPENSIVE

In the pharmaceutical industry, the common goal of all scientists, engineers, and business people is to create and develop new drugs. At least some of these drugs must be profitable enough to repay the huge costs of their development and to make up for unsuccessful drugs. Consider first the expensive path of study that followed the development of plant alkaloids into drugs, because it recurs in many other cases of medical research. A crude natural product or a synthetic chemical is obtained, purified, and screened for biological activities. In the case of natural products, some idea of what effect to look for comes from folklore. As unreliable as such traditions are, they did, and sometimes still do, suggest better biological test methods than random screening.

When the chemical structure of a compound is known, as it is for most synthetic substances, further guidance as to what biological test might be fruitful comes from comparing it with structurally similar chemicals with known biological properties. Thus, if a new test compound contained a certain ring of carbon and other elements, and if other compounds containing the same ring as a "skeleton" have lowered the blood pressure of laboratory animals, then the new compound might also lower blood pressure, and testing for this property would be in order.

The two hardest decisions for modern administrators of drug research and informed business executives alike are what specific research to start and when to stop it. Suggestions and requests for novel drug therapies usually come from consulting physicians who discuss these possibilities with physicians within the company. The pharmacologists and other experimental biologists are consulted early to decide whether they can set up a suitable test to screen for the required activity. As the understanding of the biochemistry of some diseases improves, ideas for a new drug research project increasingly arise from participating scientists, biochemists, enzymologists, and molecular pharmacologists. If the proposed program requires the isolation and inexpensive manufacture of hormones or nutritional substances (essential amino acids, vitamins), organic chemists and fermentation experts in the company will have to judge the possibility of success of these operations.

Recently, a technique called recombinant DNA (deoxyribonucleic acid) has permitted the commercial production of extremely complicated hormones and drugs, such as human insulin, by so altering the genetic mechanisms of bacteria and yeasts that they make the desired compounds. Almost all major pharmaceutical research companies have started recombinant DNA experiments and have expanded their staffs by employing geneticists and other experts in these fields.

Obviously, during the lifespan of patent protection, most of the widely used effective drugs are highly priced. Consider the cost of developing a drug through preclinical and clinical trials; this amounts to $80–90 million and this amount has to be amortized during the period protected by the patent. Since the maximum length of patent protection is twenty-two years and the patent is usually issued during the preclinical work-up (about three years), one must subtract the time of clinical testing from the remaining nineteen years. Clinical trials of average drugs take four to eight years, say six years; this leaves 16 years to recoup $80–90 million and to make a profit from which future investigations will be financed. At a modest rate of 10–12 percent of annual interest, the company has to chalk up a return of over $7 million per year just to pay off the investment and overhead and to achieve a modest 3–5 percent dividend and a nest egg for future research. Not many drugs provide such an income. Once in a while, however, certain new and revolutionary medicines score very high indeed. Hoffmann-La Roche's diazepam (Valium), an antianxiety drug, became the best-seller among all prescription drugs worldwide and maintained this position for several years. Its sales were reported to add up to $1 billion per year, but have declined now. The next best-seller was SmithKline Beckman Corporation's cimetidine (Tagamet), used principally to treat (and frequently cure) stomach and intestinal ulcers and pathologically high levels of stomach acid (hyperchlorhydria). During its peak years, its sales also may have amounted to $1 billion.

These exceptional cases bear witness to the sad fact that a large proportion of the world's population is beset with anxieties that, as is well known, are often a part of the vicious circle that leads to stomach ulcers, hence to more anxiety, and so forth. If fears of the future, of wars, economic and social pressures, and disasters, of crippling sicknesses, and of course, of inevitable death could be removed, drugs like diazepam or cimetidine would be in less demand.

Many other drugs for functional and infectious disorders have also chalked up respectable sales and profits. Derivatives of cephalosporin that are taken by mouth have often superseded injectable drugs against bacterial infections. Their sales amount to hundreds of millions of dollars. Drugs that lower the blood pressure, such as propranolol (a beta-adrenergic blocking agent), and the diuretics furosemide and hydrochlorothiazide, are in the same league, and many other examples could be cited.

Anything that sells for very large sums becomes an incentive for competitors, who try to capture a percentage of the market. After the expiration of a patent, some manufacturers and distributors of drugs will produce and promote the original drug in its generic form. Several foreign chemical companies, especially in Italy, Turkey, and other countries, now produce the raw materials of generic drugs. The purified high-quality powders or liquids are shipped to Western Europe or the U.S.A., where they are made into tablets or coated pills.

Some pharmaceutical companies watching the profitable sales of a drug by another firm prefer not to wait until the original patent has expired. They want to market a competitive product that they hope will have some advantages over the original proprietary drug. Such substances may have a different chemical structure or biological action, but all too often they are only minor modifications of the drug they imitate. Even the best patent attorney cannot foresee all the little changes a competitor might make, and the most comprehensive testing of chemical variants will still allow the chemists of another firm to sidestep the claims of a drug patent.

Some people contemptously refer to such competitive medicines as "me too" drugs, but they forget that different products with virtually the same spectrum of biological activities have one real justification. No two patients are alike in their response to a given drug. A prescribed antihistamine may only relieve one person's allergies, while others also become drowsy and sleepy when they take exactly the same drug, and these reactions will be reversed with yet another of the thirty-odd antihistaminics on the market. These differences are caused by the metabolic variations among patients and the workings of their immune defense systems. In any event, the availability of alternative similar drugs has important medical advantages, as physicians know.

MODERN DRUG DISCOVERY AND DEVELOPMENT

Today the first problem in getting a new drug for a given health problem is to make plans for the chemical and biological work. A number of options are open to the participating scientists. The oldest of these is screening by subjecting a group of likely chemicals to a biological test in which some conditions of the clinical disease are imitated in laboratory animals. The requirement for success in screening programs is to develop a suitable, reliable, repeatable, biological test that is quick and not too expensive.

These requirements are most easily met in the design of drugs to treat infectious diseases. The bacteria, protozoa, rickettsiae, and viruses are invaders foreign to the human or animal host. These organisms usually differ from higher animals in nutritional needs and internal chemical (metabolic) reactions. Thus, a chemical attack tailored to these microbes has a better-than-average chance of causing less harm to tissues and cells of the host. In addition, many disease-causing microbes (pathogens) can infect a number of hosts, including laboratory mice, rats, other rodents, etc. Thus, human and bovine tubercle bacilli infect mice; malarial parasites (*Plasmodium berghei* for mice and *P. knowlesii* for monkeys) are similar to those that cause human malarias; the human leprosy bacillus has been implanted into armadillos; and many other bacteria (staphylococci, gonococci, streptococci, etc.) thrive only too well in small laboratory animals. If a new chemical succeeds in killing such infections, or at least in stopping their growth in mice, without being too toxic to these animals, there is a good chance that it may become an antibiotic for infected humans.

The greatest difficulties in developing drugs of this type are encountered with experimental viral infections, because viruses need living cells for their life processes; they take over part of the host cells' metabolic functions and thus offer the chemotherapist or drug healer a mixed situation. Parts of the infected cells act like the virus; other parts retain the characteristics of the original cell; and these actions are hard to separate. A chemical that subdues a virus often also subdues some of the life processes of the infected cells. As one wit said, "Flu is that disease that makes you feel sick six weeks after you get well."

The situation is similar in noninfectious diseases in which the metabolism of some body cells has deteriorated. Drugs to heal such disorders must restore the functions of the diseased cells without disturbing the normal body cells that surround them. At the very least, such drugs should concentrate in the diseased organ, but not elsewhere in the body. When one considers the circulation of the blood, this is asking the near impossible, and yet it has been achieved time and again. Animal tests that mimic a human disease will often allow a drug to be selective in this manner, but the drug still will not work for humans. The reason for such failures is that no two animal species metabolize foodstuffs or foreign chemicals in exactly the same way. In some animals, a drug circulating through the blood or lymph vessels will be held up by otherwise indifferent proteins, or it may pass through membranes that form a barrier in other animals. Some drugs are attacked and destroyed by certain body chemicals in one species but not in others. All this means that the metabolism of a drug has to be determined in at least two or three species—mouse, dog, rabbit, etc.—before any predictions about its clinical behavior can be made. These obstacles must be overcome to determine whether the concentration of the drug in a body fluid—usually blood—is the same in man as in an animal in which the drug works well. These measurements, carried out by refined and sensitive chemical analyses, can help pharmacologists choose among promising drugs for clinical trials.

CLINICAL TRIALS

These form the most time-consuming, expensive, and unnerving part of the introduction of a new drug. Clinical trials are never done within the walls of the company that conducts the research, but are always farmed out to clinical pharmacologists and other specialists in internal medicine, often in university-affiliated hospitals. The company pays the bills for hospital beds, clinical apparatus, and tools; salaries of physicians, nurses, orderlies, and test volunteers; and the expenses of patients who agree to try out the new drug. When the high overhead expenses charged by most hospitals are added, the bill for clinical trials quite commonly runs to $50 million or more. After learning a drug's toxicity in several animal species, the clinical researchers must find the range of nontoxic doses in healthy volunteers, with their informed consent. The drug may be administered by injection (parenterally) or by mouth (orally). The oral dose is usually greater because of the obstacles to absorption in the stomach and intestines. The effect of the drug on body weight and functions, individual organs, and the general health of the volunteer are recorded and reported to the Food and Drug Administration. Next come gingerly trials in patients suffering from diseases that the drug is intended to benefit.

In some instances patients with a given disease may be hard to find. For example, malaria has been almost wiped out in moderate climatic zones by killing with insecticides nearly all the female *Anopheles* mosquitoes that carry this disease to people. It is therefore not practical to search for volunteer patients with malaria except in humid and relatively primitive tropical locations. In such cases, local volunteers will have to agree to be bitten by malaria-carrying mosquitoes so that the new drug may be tested on the course of their disease and, one hopes, may cure it.

It is necessary to eliminate all bias in clinical trials. To achieve this, drugs are administered by double-blind methods. Only the principal investigator will know the dosage of a drug, and which tablet or syringe actually contains the drug. Other tablets and syringes, looking completely alike, will usually contain a placebo, that is a preparation containing no medicine (often glucose sugar). Sometimes other look-alike forms may contain a different drug of known value in the disease under study. The doctors and nurses who give the drug are kept in the dark about the composition and strength of the doses so that their expectations cannot influence the patients' behavior. In this manner statistically valid comparisons of the effects of the drug can be obtained, and such comparisons are demanded by the Food and Drug Administration before approval of a new drug application is considered for general use.

There are many other aspects of clinical trials that cannot be included here, but a few inherent pitfalls follow. If effectiveness of a drug cannot be established, all trials will be stopped immediately, because giving even a slightly toxic but ineffective substance can only endanger a patient without benefitting him. On the other hand, considerable toxicity will be disregarded if the drug helps a life-threatening condition for which no other therapy is available. That is the case in some drug-resistant infections and also in cancers unless some alternative treatment (surgery, irradiation therapy) can be chosen.

While clinical trials are going on, animal experiments will be continued to determine the long-term effects of the drug on every body organ, because this cannot be done in humans within the time allotted for the original clinical trials. In the meantime also, the manufacture has to be scaled up from laboratory quantities to commercial production of kilograms or even tons of the drug. The length of time that the drug remains effective will have to be established, and the manufacture of tablets, pills, and sterile solutions for injections worked out. These are not foolproof operations, because mechanical compresssion, humidity, or heat may affect an otherwise stable compound. No organic compound is stable indefinitely, and therefore drugs should be discarded after their expiration date.

The real evaluation of a drug by the medical profession gets underway as soon as the drug is approved and becomes available for general use. In this country, concerned doctors will publish their findings in medical journals, and the Food and Drug Administration may or may not take them into account when changing its regulatory guidelines. In the United Kingdom and most European countries, physicians are required to send their observations to the agencies that control the use of drugs. Such observations are not all negative. To be sure, most physicians will report unwanted or toxic side effects, but the significance of such phenomena—nausea, rashes, malaise, headaches, etc., attributed to the drug—must be evaluated statistically and not on the basis of scattered individual cases.

The clinical trials have become a jumble of scientific and legal requirements. The Delaney Amendment to the Pure Food and Drug Act rules that no food additive that causes cancer in any animal species may be tried in humans. The pharmaceutical industry has voluntarily extended this rule to drugs and routinely, before clinical trials, tests every drug in several animal species for any increase in the numbers of cancers found. This is time-consuming and expensive, but it is necessary to avoid later litigation for malpractice. A similar situation holds for the potential ability to cause birth defects (teratogenicity) of a compound. Teratogenicity is a damage to genes. Its effects are pronounced in the early stages of fetal development and can result in death or deformed or poorly functioning offspring. A drug that is teratogenic in laboratory animals may or may not be so in human females. Teratogenicity for humans cannot be tested in controlled clinical trials because obviously a physician will not expose a pregnant patient to that risk. Such damaging properties are only discovered later, after the drug has been in general use, and in such a case the drug will be withdrawn immediately. If a drug has some beneficial activity (as with thalidomide, which was good for insomnia), it is regrettable that men of all ages and postmenopausal women must be deprived of it. However, if such drugs were available in a medicine cabinet, they could not be withheld legally from young women who do not or will not read, or who will disregard a label "not to be used by women of child-bearing age."

An additional legal burden on clinical trials is the number and frequency of the reports on effectiveness, side effects, and toxic effects of the test drug that must be submitted to the Food and Drug Administration. This unproductive paper work has alienated many clinical pharmacologists and has caused some multinational corporations to support clinical trials abroad, where the requirements are easier.

During preclinical experiments and especially during careful clinical trials, observations of new and unexpected biological activities of a test drug may be recorded. For example, the drug imipramine that was tested against psychoses revealed its ability to relieve depression during clinical trials. In the same way the diuretic (urine-producing) hydrothiazides were found to lower the blood pressure. Propranolol and other drugs called beta blockers for controlling rapid heartbeats (cardiac fibrillation) turned out to lower the blood pressure, to quiet the pain of angina pectoris, and even to reduce fluid pressure in the eye from glaucoma. In such cases, medicinal chemists will be encouraged to change the molecular structure of the compound in the hope of suppressing its original action and converting the newly discovered "side effect," to the main activity. This means, of course, going back to first base and taking the new substances through all preclinical and clinical stages. However, this is a valuable method for learning to design new drugs.

If one of the side actions of a drug is prominent enough to deserve immediate clinical application, the FDA will have to amend its approval of the use of the drug to include the newly discovered use. This often takes considerable time because evidence and paper work have to wind their way through bureaucratic channels. These delays, which deprive patients of valuable help, have been criticized. However, effectiveness and lack of toxicity at the dose levels necessary for the new activity are the overriding considerations for extending drug approval.

4

Molecular Modification of Prototype Drugs

Discovery of a totally new chemical with a novel biological activity is such a long-range gamble that the drug industry is forced into short-term efforts to furnish drugs with moderate-to-good potential value. The search for look-alike drugs is an example of this reasonable undertaking. Indeed, the majority of chemists in the pharmaceutical industry are synthesizing and studying such drugs by a process called molecular modification. Because of the importance of this work, a few explanations of their techniques are in order.

A chemist does not set out to make a drug that acts exactly like one already known, with all its advantages and disadvantages. Instead, an investigator will try to overcome the disadvantages, usually unwanted side effects and signs of toxicity. Perhaps the new substance should be more powerful so that a smaller dose can be given, presumably with fewer side effects because less drug will be present in the body.

If two different chemicals are to cause a similar effect, they will probably have to react at the same chemical positions or receptors on the target cells. For this purpose they must fit almost as snugly to these receptors. Picture a glove that fits your left hand. Another person of similar size may try on one of your gloves and find that the left hand will fit your glove, but neither your right hand nor that of your friend will fit it. In other words, a similar shape of the two biologically active molecules is required for similar biological action.

But similarity of shape is not enough. There must be some inducement for the molecules to approach the receptors and bind to them. Chemical attraction between two molecules—drug and receptor—is caused by electrons. Electrons are negatively charged and therefore are attracted to positive poles or places; they are "nucleophilic." When an electron is removed, the portion of an electrically neutral molecule that stays behind has lost a negative charge and so becomes positively charged. Such a "positive ion" then tries to become neutral and at rest by joining an electron-rich, negatively charged particle somewhere else; it is "electrophilic." Although this account is an oversimplification of chemical reactions, it may serve to illustrate some essentials of chemical similarity. In order for two different chemicals to react at the same receptor, they must have similar shapes and similar electronic behavior. This behavior is also called similar binding ability because binding comes about by joining or transfer of electrons. The similarity of binding and shapes in biologically active molecules is called bioisosterism (from the Greek: *bios* = life, *isos* = like, *stereos* = shape). Two chemically and biologically similar active compounds are bioisosteric.

Medicinal chemists have worked out a set of rules and limitations for this property, and they apply them to drugs that they want to imitate. Following these guidelines usually results in a number of similar compounds (analogs), but only a few of them are suitable for further study—a great waste of time and effort, because all the other analogs will be discarded.

Computer-minded chemists have tried to limit the numbers of almost-right compounds by measuring various properties of a set of chemicals and having the computer pit one against another. This helps occasionally and is cheaper than wasting months of laboratory time. Therefore almost all research companies have installed computers for that kind of work. On the whole, changing molecules bit by bit remains an art in which experience, luck, and clever experimentation go hand in hand with sophisticated calculations of electron clouds and shapes of molecules as determined by X-ray diffraction. It is very hard to decide how to improve upon the structure of a useful drug. To do so one has to work within the limits of shape and electrical affinity and try one's luck time and again.

The life processes of animals, including human beings, are caused and regulated by tens of thousands, perhaps more, of chemical reactions. Many kinds of body chemicals have been isolated and identified, and some of their usually multiple functions have been described. But innumerable puzzles remain. It is as if the yarn needed to make a multicolored rug had been spread on the floor, and the weaver explained that people would walk on the rug after it was made, but failed to say how the weaving and blending of the different strands would be done—perhaps he would decide details as he went along. In life, the actual interactions of the spectrum of biochemical "yarns" found in an animal organism are difficult to determine, because methods for studying them in their natural environment are very complicated.

The Harvard psychiatrist Seymour Kety has illustrated this dilemma further. A delegation of extraterrestrial beings came to visit Earth and wanted to learn what makes humans tick. They decided on a biochemical analysis of the earth creatures. A few hundred people were caught and ground up in a giant meat grinder, and the material was extracted, fractionated, and identified chemically. The Martians found dozens of amino acids, hormones, nucleosides, and many other compounds. They arranged this mixture in what they thought was a logical sequence and nodded wisely. Now we know, one of them said, how the humans composed Beethoven's Ninth Symphony, wrote Shakespeare's *Hamlet*, Goethe's *Faust*, the Koran and the Bible, and built the Golden Gate Bridge and the Taj Mahal. We are still at the same stage of interpreting life processes.

With the coming of very sensitive analytical instruments in the last forty years, scientists have been able to study ever smaller amounts of hormones, parts of the immune system, tumor-causing viruses, fragments of nucleic acids and genes, traces of metal ions and other elusive biochemicals. At first, progress was slow because the sheer learning of the new methods took years and all the difficulties that bedevil complicated new enterprises had to be ironed out. Lately the pace has speeded up, and the new methods are spreading to such fields as genetics and psychology, with startling results. Scientists are even beginning to explain such biological mysteries as memory in terms of chemical reactions.

When a drug is administered, it intrudes into this interwoven, ever-changing, and unbelievably complex array of biochemical reactions and is supposed to restore "normality," or homeostasis, the name given by the physiologist Cannon to a healthy interplay of all the factors that keep the body running smoothly. Yet using a drug is a bit like sweeping a broom through a disorganized mass of litter while trying to line up the pieces in an orderly way. The nature of homeostatic mixtures of chemicals or of their disorganized states in disease is very difficult to unravel, but now at least we know many individual chemicals in the mixtures, although many of their reactions still baffle us.

Fortunately, the individual puzzle pieces can be mentally and chemically rearranged much as molecular modifications form the basis of designing similar drugs. Molecular modification has already been applied to hundreds of products called metabolites that have been fished out of the mixture of biochemicals in living organisms. The reasoning behind these experiments is that Nature has not necessarily evolved the best chemicals for a given purpose, but often only the most chemically convenient. For example, cortisone and hydrocortisone are found among similar compounds in extracts of the outer layer or cortex of the adrenal gland. These two hormones help to counteract inflammation and arthritis, but are by no means the best substances for this purpose. By changing these molecules, medicinal chemists have synthesized similar analogs (prednisolone, dexamethasone) that are highly useful drugs with stronger and more selective action on inflammation.

Two examples of successful molecular modifications of metabolites are para-aminosalicylic acid and methyldopa. Salicylic acid was believed to support oxidation of tubercle bacilli. *para*-Aminobenzoic acid (PABA) is a general growth factor (vitamin) for bacteria that make folic acid, a product biosynthesized from PABA. By combining salicylic acid and PABA in one molecule, chemists produced a drug called para-aminosalicylic acid that has become an effective treatment for human tuberculosis.

The other example is based on an amino acid called dopa for short, which serves as a precursor for dopamine. Dopamine in turn is converted further into epinephrine (adrenaline), which causes some types of high blood pressure. A small CH_2 group was added to dopa to make methyldopa, which blocks the chemical pathway to epinephrine. This is one way to control blood pressure. In the long run, and by various methods, high blood pressure can be reduced to more normal levels.

The most successful use of modified metabolites as drugs has been to combat foreign or malignant invasive cells. Cancer cells divide in an uncontrolled, often rapid fashion. Because each new daughter cell needs a cell nucleus, nuclear material—especially DNA and RNA types of nucleic acids—must constantly be manufactured in these cells. These nucleic acids contain several basic units called purines and pyrimidines. Two of these are adenine, a purine derivative, and uracil, a pyrimidine derivative. By making a slight change in adenine, one obtains 6-mercaptopurine, which enters the chemical conveyor belt leading to a nucleic acid but, being a faulty building block, prevents the construction of a working nucleic acid and thereby of new cell nuclei.

Another example is even simpler. By synthetically exchanging one small atom of hydrogen in uracil with a not much larger atom of fluorine, one can make 5-fluoruracil, which likewise prevents DNA from functioning in forming a new cancer cell nucleus. Physicians use these two drugs as powerful "antimetabolites" for chemotherapy to treat many cancers in addition to or instead of surgery or radiation.

The chemical methods for molecular modification are also used in planning drugs to counteract metabolites. The best part of trying to develop a new metabolite antagonist, as they are called here, is that the chemist need not imitate a competitor's drug but instead uses as the starting point natural substances made by the body—a much more satisfying scientific motivation.

5

Neurohormones and Drugs That Affect the Central Nervous System

Ever since alcohol, opium, cannabis (marijuana, hashish), tobacco, and peyote began to be used by humans, medicines that alter mental states have been regarded with awe, fear, disgust, and other emotions. Some of these substances cause detachment and withdrawal or result in sleep or indifference to outside influences. For centuries surgeons used alcohol and opium to blunt the intolerable pain of amputations and other operations. Some drugs were used in religious or orgiastic rites where the participants wanted to communicate with imaginary deities or to shed restrictions taught by their societies. In lower doses than those causing drunkenness or completely drugged behavior, alcohol and marijuana improve sociability and provide a feeling of success. A sniff of ether may produce overexcitement, and barbiturates and other hypnotics sedate, making animals and humans go to sleep. Such sedative-hypnotics are thought to be the earliest drugs used for depressing brain activity. At the other end of the spectrum, cocaine, amphetamine, and to some extent, ephedrine were among the early brain stimulants that could overcome sleepiness, increase wakeful awareness, and improve the ability to perform complex tasks.

In 1867 one of the founders of organic chemistry, Adolf von Baeyer, first synthesized a laboratory curiosity called acetylcholine. He had no idea that he had described an important neurohormone. Later (1900), the American physiologist Hunt studied the effects of acetylcholine (ACh) and found that it depressed the blood pressure in laboratory animals. Because this property promised to reduce high blood pressure in humans, extensive pharmacological work followed. Two contrasting types of activity of ACh were found. One resembled that of nicotine and was called nicotinic; the other, similar to that of the mushroom poison muscarine (which had been identified as the highly toxic substance in the fly agaric, *Amanita muscaria*), was called muscarinic. Because these different properties are subdivisions of the total action of ACh, they were named cholinergic. Antispasmodic drugs such as atropine block the muscarinic component of cholinergic activities but have little impact on the nicotinic action of ACh.

Each involuntary (autonomic) muscle and gland is "wired" (innervated) by two types of nerves: the sympathetic (adrenergic), which react with norepinephrine, and the parasympathetic (cholinergic), which react with ACh. Any two nerve cells are joined by a fine network of fibers (dendrites), which are enmeshed in a junction called the synapse. Because the dendrites of one nerve cell do not touch those of the next one, a tiny space separates them. Bridging is done by a current transmitter dissolved in water droplets. In the parasympathetic nervous system, the transmitter is acetylcholine at all points; in the sympathetic nervous system, the transmitter is norepinephrine (noradrenaline), while between the tip of a sympathetic nerve and the end organ (muscle or gland) that it stimulates, the transmitter is acetylcholine.

These fundamental life processes were explained by the brilliant experiments of neuropharmacologists. Otto Löwi in 1921 discovered the role of acetylcholine, and Ulysses von Euler in 1946 determined that of norepinephrine. More recently, several other neurotransmitters have been found, especially dopamine, 5-hydroxytryptamine (5-HT, or serotonin), gamma-aminobutyric acid (GABA), and between thirty and fifty peptides (combinations of several amino acids).

Some of these compounds may not be true neurotransmitters, but only modulate links in a chain of events leading to impulse transmission across the synapse. Some of them appear to play specialized health roles, such as lifting depression by 5-HT and blunting pain by the body's own enkephalin peptides.

An electrical signal has to be amplified as it travels along a nerve, and this is accomplished by creating simple sodium, potassium, and calcium ions—that is, electrically charged atoms—from nonionized salts. In turn, the activation of these ions is performed by stepwise ionization of the transmitters and modulators just described. This is a greatly simplified picture of the way nervous impulses flow, but should suffice to guide us in discussions of drugs that stimulate, depress, or disorganize the nervous systems. Some of these drugs have freed us from age-old prejudices and have improved the treatment of mental and nervous diseases beyond the wildest expectations of only thirty years ago.

The first biochemicals recognized as neurotransmitters, ACh and norepinephrine, faced a number of hurdles initially. Norepinephrine especially was an afterthought to the discovery of epinephrine (adrenaline) at the turn of the century. Epinephrine was found in the adrenal glands, which are located at the top and back of the kidneys. The glands consist of an inner layer (the adrenal medulla) and an outer layer (the adrenal cortex). The adrenal medulla secretes epinephrine; the cortex secretes cortisone, hydrocortisone (cortisol), and many similar steroid hormones. Among a number of other functions, epinephrine constricts blood vessels, increases blood pressure, stimulates the heart, and raises the concentration of sugar in the blood. It was relatively simple to synthesize epinephrine in the laboratory. In the course of this work its slightly smaller first cousin, norepinephrine, was also prepared, although its role in nervous transmission was not explained for another forty years.

Before 1950 ephedrine and amphetamine to stimulate and barbiturates to sedate were the only important substances available to doctors for treating mental conditions. In 1952, three different drugs made their appearance and opened up the era of true therapeutic drugs in psychiatry. They were chlorpromazine, the original tranquilizer that came from France; reserpine, which originated in India and Switzerland; and meprobamate, a muscle relaxant that also allays anxieties, which hailed from New Jersey.

When most people speak of sedatives, antianxiety medicines, and antidepressants, they often call them all tranquilizers, although the three names preceding show that the substances do not fit into one category. The antipsychotic drugs, which control severe manias, should be the only ones called tranquilizers, but the term *neuroleptics* has become an accepted substitute for *antipsychotics*. Neuroleptics such as chlorpromazine do not alter consciousness or thinking, do not decrease initiative, but do make the patient less responsive to things that might harm the sense of self-worth or psyche. This definition overlooks the fact that most neuroleptics make patients at least somewhat sleepy, but that is a small price to pay for the social adjustment they bring and for smoothing out unwanted excitement and hostility as well as severe withdrawal.

The antianxiety agents (diazepam, meprobamate, etc.), also called minor tranquilizers, depress overexcitability of certain nerve paths. So do the sedative-hypnotics, although they act at different locations in the brain. The latter are used primarily by physicians to induce and maintain curative sleep. These medicines share this property with several antihistamines that have a sleep-inducing (hypnotic) side effect so strong that they have been chosen as ingredients for several over-the-counter sleep-producing medicines. Users are not told that a hangover usually awaits them the next day and that they may become uncooperative and resentful until the drug has been eliminated.

Antidepressant drugs stimulate the central nervous system's parts that control emotion and mood. This they do by preventing the absorption of certain chemicals (biogenic amines) by nerve endings and thereby freeing them for special biochemical uses. The antidepressants have also been called thymoleptics and some of them psychic energizers. Another drug—this time an inorganic one—is useful for mental disease. Lithium salts are used to blunt the manic phase of manic-depressive states (biphasic depression).

ANTIPSYCHOTIC AGENTS

The history of these and all the other important psychopharmacological drugs is an account of accidental observations, with only marginal intrusions of logic. A fancy name for this kind of development is serendipity. The only exception is reserpine, the main alkaloid of *Rauwolfia serpentina,* a shrub that grows in India and around the Pacific basin. Its pink and white blossoms decorate the southern slopes of the Himalayas. The bush was called *pagla-ka-dawa* (insanity herb) by the Sherpas; its Sanskrit name in Ayurvedic medicine was *sarpagandha.* The French botanist Plumier in 1703 called it *Rauwolfia serpentina* in honor of a sixteenth century Augsburg botanist, Leonard Rauwolf, and because its roots are snakelike. Historians have found no evidence that Rauwolf ever saw the plant or even heard of it.

As was the custom with medicinal plants of old, rauwolfia was used to treat many different conditions—in alphabetical order, cataract, cholera, epilepsy, insanity, insomnia (which may have been due to high blood pressure), and snake bite (because of the shape of its roots!). Modern Indian chemists extracted the plant and found that it was active in the treatment of high blood pressure (hypertension) and psychoses. At first nobody paid any attention to the publication of these findings in an obscure Indian journal, but twenty-five years later (1949) one of the Indian authors (Vakil) described his results in a British journal, and that started the ball rolling. Reserpine was isolated and characterized in the Ciba laboratories in Basel, and the complicated alkaloid was synthesized by Robert Woodward of Harvard University, probably the greatest organic chemist of this century.

Although reserpine has lost ground in psychiatry because of the depression that accompanies tranquilization, it is still used to treat some forms of high blood pressure. It acts by releasing several biogenic amines from nerve endings and thereby making these neurohormones available for their mood-regulating tasks.

Chlorpromazine was developed through a series of studies that started with some antiallergic (antihistaminic) drugs derived from an organic chemical called phenothiazine. As mentioned before, some antihistamines make the user sleepy. This depression of the central nervous system is a prominent side effect and not their principal activity. French chemists led by Paul Charpentier tried to separate the allergy control from the depressive effect by molecular modification. Most antihistamines of that type contain a chain of two carbon atoms connecting two nitrogen atoms, and this chain was made longer by synthesis. The resulting chemical had an amazing variety of biological activities, which made it hard to classify and to study for one activity at a time. In fact, the French called it Largactil for its "large actions." One clinician noted that it lowered the body temperature and used the compound to cool patients before heart surgery by artificial hibernation. Now, cooling the body in cold, wet sheets was a rough old method of treating raging insane patients. The new drug, chlorpromazine, was therefore given to these psychotic patients by the psychiatrist Delay in Paris, with excellent results. In this country chlorpromazine was first given gingerly as an antiemetic to counteract vomiting but was finally tested against psychoses under the trade name of Thorazine in 1954. It soon became the standard drug for treating psychotic patients.

It is not surprising that a drug with so many activities has a number of unwanted clinical side effects. The most objectionable of these are the extrapyramidal symptoms that some patients develop after prolonged treatment. These symptoms take the form of tremors similar to those in Parkinson's disease, the old "shaking palsy." This problem became the scientific driving force for trying to improve chlorpromazine by molecular modification. An estimated 10,000 similar compounds have been prepared and tested, a monumental worldwide effort that produced a dozen or so drugs now in clinical use. The most acceptable of these is thioridazine, which causes fewer Parkinson-type cases, although the symptoms could not be eliminated altogether.

An equal motivating force to modify chlorpromazine was the desire of almost every pharmaceutical firm to secure a share of the market commanded by this drug, as shown by its spectacular curative and economic results in hospitals for mental patients. Within three years after the introduction of chlorpromazine, most of these inadequately staffed, overcrowded hospitals were emptied because psychotic patients could be released and returned to their homes and useful occupations. The savings in public and private funds were enormous. Construction of new mental health facilities could be halted. The state of New York alone saved approximately two billion dollars over a seven-year period. The gain in human happiness and the joy of reunited families cannot even be estimated.

The effects of antipsychotic drugs—and also of antidepressant and antianxiety agents—changed the public's attitude toward mental disease. Regarded with superstitious fear, distrust, despair, and rejection since ancient times, psychoses and depressions are now generally recognized as functional diseases, not unlike diabetes, goiter, and other organic sicknesses that can be corrected. An attitude of kindness and understanding has replaced the horror of centuries of ignorance in clinical and personal relations with mental patients.

The feverishly competitive research on phenothiazines in the 1950s and 1960s not only resulted in new drugs but led to the invention of biological tests that provided a better comparison with human psychotic states. That meant finding behavioral tests for laboratory animals that had been given test drugs. The most common of these tests are based on what is called conditioned avoidance behavior and "learned" responses to the drug. Typically, an animal is placed in a cage with an electrically wired bottom. There is a wooden pole or a rope overhead. The animal is taught to avoid an electric shock to its feet by climbing the pole or the rope. Under the influence of an effective test drug, the escape by climbing will be delayed and the effect of a given voltage diminished. Or an animal will first be rewarded by food or drink for pressing a lever, then, when treated with a useful test drug, this learned response will be slowed. A whole battery of behavioral tests is usually employed to study the various actions of a test compound.

With such methods, it became possible to screen thousands of diverse chemicals for chlorpromazine-like reactions. From these tests emerged the butyrophenone class of antipsychotics, of which about ten are used abroad. Only one—haloperidol—has been approved in the U.S.A. Haloperidol was developed by the Belgian medicinal chemist and pharmacologist Paul A. J. Janssen through a series of chemical comparisons to other drugs, but not to chlorpromazine.

The starting point of Janssen's researches was meperidine, a morphinelike pain reliever known since the 1930s and studied in Germany before World War II. Its American proprietary name is Demerol. Janssen made a large number of substances similar to meperidine and screened them for several activities, among them the then fashionable test for conditioned avoidance. Scientists follow fashions like the rest of the world. The butyrophenones were vague and rather farfetched variations of meperidine, really not well related to that drug. They proved more potent than chlorpromazine but, unfortunately, shared with chlorpromazine the objectionable Parkinson-type reactions. Haloperidol is preferred to phenothiazine drugs by some psychiatrists but not by others.

On the chemical way to the butyrophenones, about 4,000 intermediates and analogs were prepared and screened, among them diphenoxylate, which turned out to be a useful cough supressor and worked especially well for diarrhea by relaxing the intestines. It has become a standby for travelers visiting foreign countries.

The phenothiazine drugs (chlorpromazine, thioridazine, etc.), the butyrophenones (haloperidol), and related agents are used in psychiatric practice to treat insanity and psychoses. Neuroses are not usually treated with these drugs but rather with antianxiety agents, sedatives, or by psychoanalysis.

ANTIDEPRESSANTS

Antidepressants relieve the deep depression arising from a disturbed concentration of essential chemicals (biogenic amines) in brain tissues (such as the *corpus coeruleum* and the *substantia nigra*). Depression caused by grief, personal loss, and similar temporary conditions do not respond to typical antidepressants. They can be relieved by antianxiety drugs.

In order to understand this difference, one must know a little of the physiological origin of internal (endogenous) depressions. "Normal" moods and emotions are maintained by the reactions of certain neurotransmitters at brain receptors which work much as previously explained in conducting currents from one nerve cell to the next.

Of these neurotransmitters, three biogenic amines—dopamine (DA), 5-hydroxytryptamine (5-HT), and norepinephrine (NE)—are most important. Other substances, such as small peptide hormones, may also be involved. A loss of the amines at their brain receptors can come about in two ways. One is the return of the amines into storage granules in nerve endings. These are microscopically small reservoirs that serve as amine storage bins. The other way is destruction by enzymes, primarily monoamine oxidase (MAO) and catalysts that alter these neurohormones by a chemical reaction called methylation.

The first antidepressants owed their discovery to the observation that one of the drugs for tuberculosis introduced in the 1950s caused unwanted, serious mental disturbances as a side effect. The Swiss pharmacologist Zeller became interested in this troublesome property and soon found by trial and error that the antituberculous drug iproniazid blocked the action of the MAO enzyme. Iproniazid was then tried clinically in severely depressed patients, and it successfully elevated their mood. Although it soon had to be withdrawn because it also damaged the liver, it pointed the way to the use of monoamine oxidase inhibitors as antidepressants. By blocking MAO, such compounds prevent the destruction of the neurotransmitters needed to maintain serenity.

A number of analogs and more remote relatives of iproniazid were tested, because the easiest way to achieve something is to do as someone else has done. Three of these, phenelzine, isocarboxazide, and nialamide, have survived as useful antidepressants. Screening of other assorted chemicals revealed two drugs for the same purpose. One was tranylcypromine, a novel relative of amphetamine; the other was pargyline. Pargyline also lowers the blood pressure, and the manufacturer of this drug preferred to introduce it for this lucrative use.

Tranylcypromine is a potent antidepressant. This and many other MAO blockers cause erratic changes in blood pressure if the patient is on an uncontrolled diet. The drugs prevent the destruction of tyramine, a widely distributed dietary substance that drives up the blood pressure. It occurs in cheeses such as cheddar, Stilton, and Camembert and in beer, bananas, canned figs, and red wines. Patients using MAO blockers are warned not to consume such foods. Human nature being what it is, such a prohibition can be completely enforced only in a hospital.

Pargyline and tranylcypromine are among the first drugs whose mode of action is fully understood at the enzyme level. Both form known compounds with MAO that change the enzyme so that it can no longer break down (oxidize) the neurotransmitter. In a way, the enzyme commits suicide by these chemical reactions. The two drugs are therefore spoken of as suicide-enzyme inhibitors.

Recently chemists have learned of another way that MAO blockers affect the fate of neurotransmitters. They slow down the return of these biogenic amines into storage spaces in nerve endings, although not as efficiently as imipramine and other tricyclic antidepressants, but they increase this action when given together with these drugs. Tranylcypromine has also been used as a drug for Parkinsonism.

The early tricyclic antidepressants had three rings of atoms in their structure, hence the name. They were conceived by R. Kuhn in Switzerland as variants of certain tranquilizers and were tested as such, but they behaved unexpectedly as antidepressants. The two standard-bearers of this class are imipramine and amitriptyline. As mentioned above, they maintain the neurotransmitters at nerve endings by preventing those biogenic amines from returning to their reservoirs.

Recently, it has been reported that desipramine, a metabolic product of imipramine, relieves the symptoms of addiction to cocaine. Imipramine has also been found useful in preventing bedwetting.

ANTIANXIETY AGENTS

Anxiety is an uneasy state of emotions akin to fear. It is a response to various disquieting environmental stimuli and is best treated by removal of such worrisome factors. If that cannot be done, an antianxiety drug may be prescribed. In fact, anxiety about other symptoms usually drives patients to see a physician, and such drugs will often be the first aid in setting the patient on the road to recovery.

It is hard to devise tests for animals that will correspond to human anxiety. Every time a laboratory animal is picked up and handled, it will be anxious, because it regards the researcher as a danger. But the symptoms of animal anxiety cannot be judged and compared, because animals cannot verbalize their fears and feelings. Therefore, other actions of drugs, such as muscle relaxation, increased or slowed heartbeats and breathing, and reduction of twitching responses to unpleasant stimuli, have become part of a battery of tests designed to screen antianxiety compounds.

Conventional wisdom claims that one cannot be anxious and relaxed at the same time. Fortunately, it is easy to measure muscle relaxation, and therefore antianxiety agents had their origin in drugs that relax skeletal muscles. Frank M. Berger pioneered in screening compounds for this quality, and selected a simple drug, mephenesin, as his prototype. Over 1,200 compounds were tested before the best, meprobamate, was chosen for in-depth clinical study. Synthesized by B. J. Ludwig, this drug has become a widely prescribed antianxiety pill.

Berger named meprobamate "Miltown" for the New Jersey town he lived in at that time. He was president of Carter Laboratories, which had previously profited from the sale of Carter's Little Liver Pills. When meprobamate came along, the company had no manufacturing facilities and turned to a larger firm, Wyeth Laboratories, for a cooperative agreement. Wyeth agreed to make meprobamate for Carter on condition that they could market part of it under their own trade name, Equanil. There are stories of patients who had taken Miltown but complained that it did not help their anxieties. The physician then changed the prescription to Equanil, and the grateful patients reported glowing success with the "new" drug. They did not know that both medicines had been made in the same batch and divided by the two companies. This illustrates some of the difficulties of treating psychosomatic disorders in which the mind upsets the body.

The commercial success of meprobamate stimulated many other pharmaceutical companies to search for similar drugs. There were not many leads, and therefore all kinds of compounds were screened in the battery of tests that Berger had published. The road to the benzodiazepines, which were destined to become the standard bearers among antianxiety agents, began in these screening experiments.

Leo H. Sternbach worked at a Polish university after 1930 on some organic chemicals that were thought to contain a ring of carbon, nitrogen, and oxygen atoms, but the methods for proving this structure were inadequate then. The work was stopped, and later Sternbach was lucky enough to emigrate from Poland and find a job as a research chemist with the large New Jersey pharmaceutical firm Hoffmann-LaRoche, Inc. After a while, he was encouraged to spend part of his time on any subject he liked, so he picked up his unfinished old studies. With the modern instruments available, he then found that the earlier chemical analysis was wrong, and the compounds had a different structure. A few were tested but proved uninteresting, and the project was abandoned.

In May 1957, the laboratory was cleaned and a leftover vial of one untested compound was taken off the shelf. Because it had not yet been screened, it was sent to Dr. Lowell O. Randall, who tested it for meprobamatelike relaxing activity. The compound was so successful that clinical trials seemed indicated.

The drug, called chlordiazepoxide (later Librium), still had an adventurous fate ahead. Today, the chemical structure of a compound is ordinarily well known before biological testing is begun. If it turns out to be biologically interesting, chemists can make variants for patent claims and can also explore whether any of them might be more powerful or more suitable. Here, however, was a drug destined to become an excellent one for reducing anxiety yet its chemistry was not understood. A strange and unexpected chemical reaction had occurred during its synthesis, and it took months before that could be explained. Only then could molecular modification begin.

These modifications soon furnished a whole string of "-azepams" that were improvements in several ways over Librium. Most important was a simpler one called diazepam, which, under the proprietary name of Valium, became the most widely prescribed of all medications and remained at the top of this best-seller list for several years. It is a good antianxiety agent. Another variant is flurazepam, which, under the name Dalmane, has become one of the drugs most widely prescribed for insomnia. It also helps to overcome jet lag.

SEDATIVE-HYPNOTICS

The word *hypnotic* comes from the name of the Greek god of sleep, Hypnos. Before people or animals go to sleep, they get drowsy, and before that they become calm. There is a steady transition from wakefulness to sedation to the various stages of sleep. Different drugs lead to intermediate stages or all the way beyond REM (rapid eye movement) sleep. Scopolamine produces twilight sleep; phenobarbital, deep sleep.

Millions of people suffer from insomnia for a variety of environmental or internal reasons. Millions of others think they cannot sleep, although in reality they are asleep much of the time most nights. Many seek sleep through the aid of drugs at least occasionally. The frequent advertisements of sleep aids on television bear witness to the need and profitability of such drugs. Ten or twenty years ago most of the over-the-counter hypnotics contained scopolamine; today the active ingredient is usually diphenhydramine, an antihistamine that blocks the H-1 receptor and has a strong component of antispasmodic and sedative (anticholinergic) activity.

The best known older hypnotics are the barbiturate drugs. Barbituric acid was first synthesized by von Baeyer in 1864, when he was an assistant at the University of Ghent in Belgium. The name arose from a Miss Barbara, a friend of von Baeyer, and from the fact that the substance is made from urea. Another version of the name connects it with St. Barbara, a military patron saint. Eighteen years later, a different derivative was synthesized in another laboratory and tried out by J. von Mering as a hypnotic in animals. The famous chemist Emil Fischer, collaborating with von Mering at that time, was going on a trip from Berlin to Italy in a sleeping car. He took some diethylbarbiturate so that he could sleep, and woke up in the Italian city of Verona, where the unhappy love affair of Romeo and Juliet took place. Therefore Fischer called the drug Veronal.

In 1912 a simple synthesis of phenobarbital was published. This powerful drug sedates or puts to sleep, depending on the dose. Later Hauptman recognized it as an effective anticonvulsant drug for epilepsy. It is still used very widely.

Two American chemists, Horace Shonle and A. Moment, then improved the chemistry of barbiturates to the point that most imaginable derivatives could be manufactured inexpensively. Such representative drugs as amobarbital and secobarbital now became available to bring sleep slowly or quickly and maintain it for three hours, six hours, etc. Next, some sulfur derivatives such as thiopental revealed the ability to produce general anesthesia for a short time when injected into a vein. The short action comes from the ease with which these compounds are metabolized and deactivated.

Many persons who have slept well after taking one of the common barbiturates sleep almost as well a second night. The chemical reason for this is that these drugs are soluble in fats and other fatlike lipids. After acting on the brain for a while, they are swept into the blood and stored in the body fat. Later, the circulating blood moves them back to the brain, where they resume their sleep-producing activity the next evening. This cycle ends only when all the drug has been broken down and eliminated.

BRAIN STIMULANTS

The neurotransmitters such as dopamine and 5-HT are essential to maintain the mood and normal emotions. They share this "tonic" property with several similar compounds, both natural and synthetic. As previously mentioned, the alkaloid ephedrine, from the desert shrub, *Ephedra vulgaris*, stimulates the brain's cerebral cortex. This plant's activity has been known in China for thousands of years. When the modern pharmacologist K. K. Chen was demonstrating this property to a class of medical students, he dosed a dog with ephedrine, and the class watched the increasing restlessness of the animal in a jiggle cage. After the students had filed out, Chen, as an afterthought, measured the dog's blood pressure and found it above normal. It then occurred to him that ephedrine's chemical structure is very similar to those of the amines that raise blood pressure by constricting blood vessels.

Several substances with chemistry similar to that of ephedrine were known and could be expected to give similar results. One of them, even simpler than ephedrine, had been synthesized in Rumania in 1887 but had been forgotten. After Gordon A. Alles prepared it again and tested it, he found that it was a good vasoconstrictor and a strong brain stimulant. The compound, named amphetamine, opened up nasal passages that had been narrowed by swollen blood vessels. It also became the standard drug for people who had to keep their attention on their work, as in driving trucks and piloting aircraft, and who had to overcome tiredness. It is interesting that amphetamine consists of two closely related substances, but only one of them, dextroamphetamine, produces the drug's desired effects. Because dextroamphetamine also overcomes emotional sluggishness, it has been widely used as a way to reduce overweight. People gain weight by overeating, often because of unhappy, lonely, or unsatisfying experiences. By overcoming such depressed feelings, dextroamphetamine helps them to stop stuffing themselves and thereby to lose unwanted pounds. A similar medicine, phenylethanolamine, is used for the same purpose.

A derivative of amphetamine that contains an extra CH_2 group in the amine portion is called methamphetamine; it is about as active as amphetamine and serves primarily as a brain stimulant. After the defeat of Japan in 1945, young Japanese had to take whatever jobs they could find, both during the day and at night. Many turned to methamphetamine to overcome sleep while on duty, because the drug was freely available without prescription. Soon many instances of frightening psychoses were traced to methamphetamine, and prolonged use of amphetamine also caused such problems. From a psychiatrist's point of view, these drug-induced psychoses became opportunities to study abnormal behavior under controlled conditions because the psychoses closely resembled several human mental diseases. It is different and more frightening when deluded young and older offbeat characters purposely take amphetamine in order to become psychotic. This problem of sick, sociological drug abuse has not yet been brought under control.

Nor is it yet possible to devise a drug that stimulates the cortex of the brain without inviting abuse. Boredom starts this abuse in those who mistakenly believe that removal of some uncomfortable symptoms will improve the underlying condition. The same story has been repeated ominously with cocaine, which also stimulates the central nervous system. Authorities can try to prevent illegal synthesis of drugs like amphetamine that require some skill to make, but it is almost impossible to control the simple extraction in water of coca leaves in poor South American countries where the economy depends on immense profits from smuggling tons of cocaine into developed countries with a free currency. The fact that their cocaine is never really pure and usually the volume is increased by substances that may be harmful does not bother these unlawful operators or those that distribute the cocaine locally.

LITHIUM

Lithium salts occur naturally in seawater and many mineral springs. Lithium urate, the lithium salt of uric acid, is, at its higher pH, more soluble in water than uric acid, which is a normal minor end product of the metabolism of nitrogen (purine) products. Patients suffering from gouty arthritis produce more uric acid than healthy individuals, and the insoluble excess is deposited as crystals in their joints. Such patients benefit from drinking lithium salt solutions because they can then excrete lithium urate and thereby decrease their gouty deposits. For this reason affluent gouty patients used to drink lithium-containing water at elegant spas, although sometimes the vacation itself and the company of secretaries or young admirers may have contributed as much to their recovery as the lithium diet. In any event, lithium therapy has had a long history, so anybody inventing a new use for lithium could bypass the time-consuming study required by the Food and Drug Administration's regulations.

The Australian psychiatrist John F. J. Cade, who studied manic-depressive illness in 1948, reasoned that abnormally high concentrations of some product in the body might cause this condition. He also felt that too low concentrations of such a substance might be the origin of melancholia, the old name for severe depression. He analyzed the urine of manic-depressive patients but could not find an unusual excretion product. Nevertheless, when the patients' urine was injected into guinea pigs, they died from fatal convulsions at one third of the deadly dose of normal human urine. So something in the urine from manic-depressives must have been more toxic to the animals. In a roundabout way this toxicity was attributed to uric acid. The investigators intended to prove this idea by adding uric acid to normal urine, which should have made it more toxic. But uric acid was too insoluble to test and therefore the more soluble lithium salt was used. To their surprise, lithium urate decreased the toxicity of urine. Then when lithium carbonate was studied alone, without urine, the animals became tranquilized. This finding was an open invitation to try lithium salts for mental patients. Schizophrenic and chronic psychotic depressive patients did not respond, but manic patients improved so much that they could be discharged from the hospital.

What does such a simple alkali ion as lithium do to suppress manic episodes? Recent studies have shown that the amounts of some fundamental hormones of metabolism such as cyclic adenosine monophosphate (*c* AMP) and inositol phosphate change under the influence of a lithium ion. These changes may account for lithium's power.

DRUGS THAT EVOKE PSYCHOSES

When early man tried out every kind of food he could find in fields and forests, he encountered mushrooms and other plants that made him feel peculiar. Later on, brews stewed from such vegetation produced similar feelings. This happened in Central and South America, in India and in Siberia, and probably all over the earth. In that way primitive people learned about plants that would raise their moods to unexpected heights or throw them into depths of fear and despair that they believed was punishment for toying with the secrets of Nature. For better or for worse they experienced strange visions they had not experienced before and glimpsed unknown insights into their "souls." In the language of today's drug abusers, they had good trips or bad trips. We must admire their persistent searching to find such plants among the inexhaustible variety of the vegetable kingdom.

Priests and witch doctors of old soon gathered these plants for their own purposes. They used them themselves and gave them to their followers at times to induce detachment but also religious frenzy or abject fear of their deities. The plants and their decoctions were also used in celebrations, to cause stupor or drunkenness, warlike excitement, and indifference to danger. In English-speaking countries the drugs contained in these plants are sometimes called psychedelic, meaning mind-manifesting. Since some of the effects they produce resemble serious mental conditions or psychoses, the name psychotomimetics is used for the group. The drugs change perception and mood, disturb the autonomic nervous system that controls normal mood, and in high doses, often cause hallucinations. Obviously physicians want to avoid these reactions, which are regarded as unwanted and feared side effects. Such drugs are therefore not used to treat patients.

We know now that natural products from the plant kingdom—and a few animal sources such as toad skins—are not the only sources of mind-tampering drugs. Many synthetic compounds, spearheaded by heroin and LSD, behave the same way. These compounds have given "drugs" such a bad name that many people overlook the value of most drugs for entirely different medicinal purposes. This negative reaction comes from the unhappiness, misery, crime, and death that have resulted when psychotomimetics are abused. Millions of young and old folk all over the world have fallen into this trap from which addiction and personality weakness often bar their escape.

Other drugs that have clinical uses but also have pronounced depressive or stimulatory side effects are excluded from this discussion because, although they are abused by unbalanced persons, their medicinal value outweighs these unfortunate occurrences. Among these drugs are morphine, atropine, scopolamine, their derivatives, and other potent analgesics and sleep inducers. All are useful medicines with side effects that are not too pronounced when used briefly. Prolonged use, however, may lead to dependence.

One of the oldest psychotomimetic drugs was soma, a concoction of unknown botanical origin used in India thousands of years ago. Sanskrit manuscripts say that it made one feel like a god. Similarly, ancient religious oracles and cults like the ones at Delphi and Eleusis in Greece drugged priestesses to visionary incoherence.

The hemp plant, *Cannabis sativa*, dates back at least to the time before Herodotus (2500 B.P.), who wrote that the Scythians on the Caspian Sea used it for self-intoxication. The crusaders encountered hashish in the Middle East made from cannabis. It was used by terrorists sent on missions of assassination. The name *hashish* means assassinate. This drug spread to high society in Europe as a means of escaping boredom, and its sinister threat culminated in this country around 1955, when millions of younger men and women began to smoke the resin of the plant. A more diluted version is called marijuana. It is not a narcotic-hallucinatory drug, but it depresses the brain, causing intellectual indifference, ineffectiveness, listlessness, and loss of productivity. Prolonged use can destroy positive personality traits. The ease of growing and harvesting hemp and the ability of Colombian, South American, and South Asian smugglers to export marijuana to America and Europe has made control of this drug virtually impossible.

The mind-affecting constitutents of cannabis are the tetrahydrocannabinols. When isolated, these compounds produce a peculiar sedation of the central nervous system at very low doses. They have helped some asthmatics and have quelled nausea for some taking anticancer drugs. Fiber from hemp is used in making certain kinds of rope.

Central America has supplied more mind-upsetting plants than any other part of the world, probably because Mexican and Peruvian jungles have been more accessible than African or Malayan tropical regions until recent times. Also the Aztecs, Otomacs, and South American Indians as well as those of New Mexico and Arizona have kept up religious cults and ceremonies in which plants play a role despite centuries of attempts to convert them to various Christian sects. This type of social culture has helped botanists to locate sources of such plants.

One of the first magic drugs discovered in Mexico and the American Southwest was *Lophophora williamsii*, also called *Anhalonium lewinii*. The parts of this spherical cactus above ground (mescal buttons) contain a number of alkaloids related to dopamine. The Indians prepare a drink from the cactus called peyote or peyotl. The drink itself, as well as mescaline and other alkaloids isolated from the cactus, have powerful mental effects and produce vivid color visions. Mescaline is a totally disorienting drug that causes long-lasting and frightening psychotic episodes. Physicians can bring them under control slowly with tranquilizing (neuroleptic) drugs. Mescaline and many of its chemical cousins have been repeatedly synthesized and tested.

Another plant still used by several Mexican tribes is ololiuqui, a herb with long white flowers and round seeds. Botanically it is called *Rivea corymbosa*, but it has a number of common names: snake plant, herb of the Virgin, and many others. The crushed seeds, or an alcoholic beverage prepared from them, induce delirium, visions, satanic hallucinations, or a narcotic type of sleep not unlike twilight sleep. The psychotomimetic substances in this plant are ergot alkaloids. Such compounds had been previously isolated from ergot, a mold growing on rye. Rye bread contaminated with ergot caused havoc in the Middle Ages in Europe, ranging from epidemics of abortions from uterine contractions to hallucinations called Saint Vitus' dance (chorea). Albert Hofmann, a Swiss biochemist, cleared up the chemistry of the new and different alkaloids from ololiuqui.

A plant called *teonanacatl* ("sacred mushroom") was regarded as a god by Mexican Indians and as the devil by Christian missionaries after the conquest of Mexico by Cortez. This mushroom contains two compounds that affect the mind, psilocin and psilocybin. Chemically they are related to the neurohormone 5-HT (serotonin). Chemists have synthesized these fairly simple compounds, and psychiatrists have tried to use them as aids to psychoanalysis and psychotherapy. The very ancient cult of the mushroom is based on colorful and unreal visions that occur as the mushroom is eaten.

Indians of the Western Amazon basin brewed a magic potion they called ayahuasca, caapi, or yajé. It is made from plants of the *Banisteriopsis* and *Tetrapterys* genera, which contain toxic alkaloids. The same alkaloids occur in a plant *(Peganum harmala)* that grows in northern steppes; its seeds were used in Arabian medicine to treat worms and to promote sweating. The harmala alkaloids are powerful blockers of the enzyme MAO, but probably are not responsible for the mental effects of the parent plants.

In the Orinoco basin, the seeds of some members of the pea family *(Piptadenia)* are ground, mixed with lime, and used widely like tobacco snuff under the name of *yopo*. Men and boys will blow the snuff into each other's nostrils through a forked tube made of chicken bones. Indian witch doctors use it to inspire prophecy and clairvoyance. *Piptadenia* contains several chemically simple indole alkaloids, among them bufotenin, which is also found in the skin of poisonous toads. The most dangerous of these substances is dimethyltryptamine, which is highly psychotomimetic. Because it is related to tryptamine, a normal biogenic amine of brain metabolism, and can be made biologically from this compound, some people think that schizophrenia perhaps results from the presence of dimethyltryptamine as a faulty metabolic product in man.

LSD, or LSD-25, is chemically named *d*-lysergic acid diethylamide tartrate. It is the most powerful and most specific psychotomimetic known. It is a synthetic compound, made by laboratory procedures, and—alas—has been at one time or another one of the most widely abused mind-altering drugs. Other amides of lysergic acid occur in the old Mexican magic plant ololiuqui and in ergot. LSD-25 was the result of standardized practice in medicinal chemistry.

The ergot alkaloids are complex derivatives of *d*-lysergic acid that have, among other properties, a uterus-contracting (oxytocic) effect that can be of use in obstetrics. Albert Hofmann in Basel, Switzerland, was given the task of modifying the structure of these compounds and testing their "cousins" for probable biological uses. He made many derivatives, one after another. The diethylamide was number 25. It was tested and, as expected, contracted the uterus of laboratory animals. It also strongly excited them.

At that point Dr. Hofmann became sick, dizzy, and restless in the laboratory, so he went home, lay down, and had what we would now call an LSD trip. It lasted for two hours, and he tried to figure out what had caused it. The last thing he had done was to prepare LSD-25; therefore, he suspected that he might have inhaled a bit of this crystalline powder. Three days later he tried to confirm his suspicion by taking one quarter of a milligram of LSD by mouth. He barely got home after that and had a really "bad trip." His family called a doctor, who stayed with him during the crisis. This experience is not hard to explain today: the effective dose of LSD in humans is less than 0.05 milligram, but poor Hofmann took five times that much. LSD is five to ten thousand times more active than mescaline and one to two hundred times more active than psilocybin from mushrooms. Its effects and dosages were confirmed in volunteers, including graduate students of the University of Basel, who still remember their experiences with a shudder.

Since the first days of the research on the classical mind-altering drugs, many other substances have been found that cause profound psychic changes. Almost all of them have side effects on the autonomic nervous system, and therefore the mental effects are accompanied by changes in heart rate, intestinal irregularities, difficulties in breathing, abrupt changes in blood pressure, etc. This all adds up to making persons very sick who set out only to "expand their minds" without understanding or believing the horrors and pains that result from taking these drugs of ill repute.

The newer horror drugs have chemical names that the users, often school dropouts, cannot pronounce, so they give them an assortment of alphabet-soup initials, which are also used to refer to them in the press and on TV. They are compounds made experimentally that have been smuggled out of research laboratories. In one case a drug had been tested as a general anesthetic before it was appropriated by abusers.

Some of these newer agents have been called synthetic heroin or designer drugs, although they are chemically unrelated to heroin and have not been designed. Two of them were side products in the manufacture of the analgesic meperidine. Others are synthetic compounds tried out by addicts in the hope that they might give them a new mental high. The most dangerous of these materials are 3-methylfentanyl and MDMA, a relative of methamphetamine. Both produce dangerous damage to the general health of the users and cause heroinlike addiction at unbelievably low doses.

These tragic experiences with the abuse of drugs raise questions of what can be done to curb abuse and whether it should be punished or allowed to disappear like other manifestations of a temporary culture. In considering whether drug abuse should be controlled and prevented, a detached scientific point of view will require judging each situation on its own merits or demerits rather than lumping unlike problems together indiscriminately. The abuses of heroin, cocaine, and marijuana can serve as examples. Heroin is an addictive narcotic; cocaine is an addictive stimulant; marijuana is a nonaddictive minor depressant of the central nervous system, with no actions that reach into the narcotic stage. Heroin causes an uncompromising craving for renewal of the narcotic dose; it is unreasonably expensive, its price being driven up by criminal suppliers and distributors who should be punished unmercifully. This holds true also for cocaine merchants and smugglers, although the addicted victims present a picture different from heroin addicts. Cocaine addicts can quit only with difficulty, but without the dread withdrawal symptoms of the morphine-heroin type. Marijuana users can quit most easily, without any more physical discomfort than that felt by chronic tobacco smokers of coffee drinkers. At the bottom of the failure to stop using this drug is psychological weakness and lack of stamina—insufficient will to lead a drug-free life. Heroin withdrawal requires medical assistance; marijuana withdrawal requires a strong personality. Cocaine withdrawal is between these two.

No legislation will prevent people from experimenting with drugs, not even in a police state. Exploring strange life situations, revolting against parental authority, and experimenting with sex and drugs has been going on for thousands of years. We happen to live near the crest of a wave of drug abuse, as has happened before in other times and places. The danger is that widespread drug abuse—apart from its criminal aspects—may lead to lassitude, social indifference, loss of initiative, and other factors that damage the virility of a civilization. China before Mao had sunk into a state of lowered stamina, not only because of undernourishment of the population, but because of widespread use of opium and hashish and the ensuing impoverishment of the users and their families. The Roman Empire crumbled perhaps because malaria weakened many of its peoples, but more likely because of drug abuse. These examples should be a warning to Americans, who—because of their wealth and geographical nearness to drug-producing countries—are the easiest target for drug dealers. It will take superhuman wisdom guided by clinical psychologists and experts in public health to make a dent in drug dependence and abuse by individuals.

ANTICONVULSANTS

The anticonvulsant or antiepileptic drugs are chemically similar to sleep-producing hypnotics. They also sedate the brain, although usually less so than the standard hypnotics. They control epilepsy by preventing or stopping the sudden bursts of electrical discharges between nerve cells in the brain that are characteristic of epileptic attacks and lead to convulsions. Some minor epilepsies produce only a dreamlike momentary unconsciousness (petit mal), while grand mal epilepsy results in generalized convulsions and loss of consciousness for an appreciable time. The explanation of epilepsies as faulty electrical discharges in the brain has not removed fear, but has done away with persistent superstitions that accused epileptics of harboring evil spirits that had to be exorcised. Saints and witches of old were often afflicted by epilepsy and were persecuted as heretics or as possessed by the devil.

Animal tests for anticonvulsant activity are relatively simple and have served to stimulate research on antiepileptic drugs, the first of which, introduced clinically in 1911, was phenobarbital. Molecular modification led to several similar products (primidone, mephobarbital, etc.), each of which has certain advantages and disadvantages. One disadvantage is their cost. Epileptic patients must protect themselves from convulsions for the rest of their lives, and an inexpensive drug such as phenobarbital may be preferred for this reason. A chemical analog, phenytoin (diphenylhydantoin), followed phenobarbital twenty-six years later and is said to cause less sleepiness during the day. Each anticonvulsant counteracts a different array of electrical discharges, so the most valuable of these drugs will prevent a variety of epileptic convulsions. Some of these drugs are more suitable for epileptic children. In recent years some chemically novel anticonvulsants have been discovered by screening, the most notable being valproic acid, a very simple organic chemical. These compounds affect the metabolism of brain chemicals such as gamma-aminobutyric acid (GABA), which may account for their effects.

DRUGS FOR PARKINSONISM

In 1817, James Parkinson described a disease, *paralysis agitans*, in his "Essay on the Shaking Palsy." This disease, which now bears his name, has a phase of tremors and abnormal movements and another one of rigidity. Parkinsonism is characterized, perhaps caused, by the almost complete lack of the neurohormone dopamine in certain brain regions (*corpus striatum* and *substantia nigra*). Parkinsonism is therefore a deficiency disease. Clearly, replacement of dopamine in these tissues might alleviate the symptoms of the disease. Getting dopamine into the brain is a problem however.

The plastic, spongy material of the brain and the spinal cord consists mostly of lipids, which are water-insoluble substances similar to fats. The main difference between brain tissue and other tissues is that although permeated by watery channels, brain tissue is not easily accessible to acid or basic compounds. It behaves as if it were enclosed in a capsule, which is called the blood-brain barrier. Only neutral substances can get through this layer of minute blood vessels and lipids. Dopamine is basic (alkaline) and cannot pass the barrier, but the more neutral precursor from which it is made in body tissues can pass. This precursor is called dopa. In the brain, but also in other tissues, dopa loses carbon dioxide and becomes dopamine, which is needed to prevent parkinsonian tremors. Large doses of dopa have to be taken in order to get a small amount through the blood-brain barrier. This overdose leads to side effects. Most of the drug loses carbon dioxide through the action of an enzyme before getting into the brain. In order to prevent this reaction, another drug is taken with the dopa to help it survive intact until it is absorbed into the brain.

Symptomatic relief from the tremors and muscle spasms of the disease can be provided by natural and synthetic antispasmodic drugs and by certain antihistamines that also block acetylcholine. The antiviral agent amantadine also improves the tremors; some antidepressant inhibitors of monoamine oxidase achieve the same result.

Similar tremors also occur as side effects when patients with mental illness are treated with antipsychotic drugs. These symptoms can be abolished by some of the anticholinergic agents.

Parkinsonism is only one of many degenerative diseases that may develop at any age, but are most prevalent in older patients. Since drugs have cured many infections that used to kill the young, the world's population is statistically older than in the past. Therefore, more of these diseases of aging have moved to the center of medical interest.

Of course the best way to evade degeneration would be to stay physiologically young much longer. Many ways have been suggested to achieve this, but none of them has remained unchallenged. Following some of these ideas and hunches, medicinal scientists have tested various chemicals for their ability to stabilize the metabolism and slow down physiological deterioration. They include substances that counteract faulty synthesis of proteins by preventing errors in the genetic information that controls formation of protein in the body. One of these chemicals is the local anesthetic and heart drug procainamide. Several rejuvenating clinics in Rumania and Switzerland specialize in injecting procaine into gullible individuals, promising them renewed youthful vigor. More to the point is the use of substances (vitamins D, E, carotene) that are known to prevent oxidation of certain (unsaturated) nutrients. The oxidized materials almost certainly contribute to malignancies and cell destruction.

Aging may also involve crosslinking of proteins (especially collagen), which increases the size of fibers and causes local or generalized tissue toughening. Some experimental drugs counteract this process in rats or mice. Production of fibrous plaques in the brain may be the cause of Alzheimer's disease. In turn, a decrease of a neurotransmitter, acetylcholine, may be involved in this affliction of forgetfulness and disorientation.

Alzheimer's disease has been studied intensively in recent years; it used to be attributed to premature or progressive senility. No useful drug for this degenerative disorder has been discovered as yet. As everybody knows, hormones control aging, and many attempts have been made to restore lagging hormonal output by giving replacements especially of testosterone and estrogens, but the results are confusing.

6

Drugs for the Relief from Pain

Pain is the most aggravating manifestation of disease, and ever since the dawn of recorded history, humans have tried to lessen, blunt, and avoid pain in all its forms. Psychological persuasion, diverting attention from painful stimuli, can go only so far in decreasing minor pain. The best way to stop pain is to remove its cause, whether through the healing of injured tissue, the cure of an infection, or surgical or radiological treatment of damaged organs. When radical treatment is undesirable, patients will try to decrease aches and pains through the use of drugs. The old Greek name for pain was *algēsis*, and chemicals that counteract pain are called analgesics or analgetics.

As in most other types of medicines, the early analgesics were crude natural products, mostly botanical or concoctions made from them by primitive methods of extraction. Opium and products of plants growing in temperate zones such as the bark of willow trees were among the first to be used. Opium is made by cooking the juice of unripe Oriental poppies to a dark tarry mass, which is powdered and can then be smoked in long pipes. It brings a feeling of well-being followed by forgetfulness and sleep, and helps to wipe out pain. This feeling of euphoria or well-being is even more pronounced from morphine, the extracted and purified main alkaloid of the oriental poppy. Morphine relieves severe pain from operations, accidents, and battle wounds, but it has the other undesirable actions mentioned earlier.

Codeine, which also occurs in opium but is manufactured in one simple step from morphine, is only one tenth as analgesic as morphine but can overcome medium to low-grade pain. It is less addictive than morphine. It also suppresses the cough reflex and is still incorporated in some cough medicines, although the less constipating, synthetic drug dextromethorphan has largely replaced it for this purpose.

Most notorious of the many hundreds of derivatives of morphine is heroin, made in a textbook operation from morphine in one step. It rapidly causes dependence that, as previously mentioned, is particularly hard to shake. The drug has to be injected to be active, and impure samples cause infections and other organic damage.

Two synthetic analogs of morphine are meperidine and methadone, both widely used to dampen pain. Methadone is also substituted for heroin to slowly wean addicts away from heroin. Both meperidine and methadone were designed by German industrial chemists to control spasms, and their power to control pain was later discovered by screening. Another widely used, moderately powerful analgesic is propoxyphen.

How the brain perceives pain and how powerful analgesics work are questions that have intrigued generations of scientists. In the early 1970s the British biochemist Hughes discovered several small and medium-sized proteinlike compounds that were named enkephalins from the Greek "within the head." These substances are short-lived but strong painkillers when injected into laboratory animals. The enkephalins are made in body cells from larger peptides called endorphins (endo = inside, + (m)orphines) whenever the need for pain relief arises. They account for the fact that people often feel little pain at first from accidents or wounds. It appears that the action of potent analgesics is conveyed to the brain by these natural peptides. Because the enkephalins are also found in portions of rat spinal cords close to nerve tissues containing norepinephrine, a connection between these two types of neurotransmitters has been suggested. Attempts to modify the enkephalins for use in controlling human pain for any length of time have been unsuccessful.

Acupuncture, the ancient oriental method of relieving pain or preventing the onset of surgical pain by inserting needles or pressing at specific places is believed by some to activate the endorphin-enkephalin system in the central nervous system and thereby to produce a profound analgesia. This theory has not been proven.

None of the strong painkillers can be obtained without a prescription. The many side effects, particularly the danger of addiction, require that they be used only when absolutely necessary to control severe pain. Many patients who suffer lesser pains can obtain mild analgesics in any drug store without a prescription. If such pains are caused by rheumatism or arthritic inflammation, as is often the case, both the old and the modern antiinflammatory drugs give very effective relief.

ANTIINFLAMMATORY AGENTS

There are two broad classes of drugs that control the hot, painful swelling of inflammation, steroidal and nonsteroidal. The steroidal agents are more effective, but also have more side effects. Therefore, they are prescription drugs. Many recently discovered nonsteroidal substances that sooth inflammation are too new to be offered as over-the-counter medicines and also require prescriptions. The older, nonsteroidal medicines—led by aspirin and followed by acetaminophen, best known as Tylenol—are the active ingredients of almost all the "pain and fever" medicines sold in the United States. In other countries several derivatives of pyrazolinone are popular, although frequent blood changes are attributed to these drugs. Ibuprofen, another effective substance for moderate pain, is now also available without prescription.

Aspirin was an old compound when the pharmacologist H. Dreser introduced it to reduce fever and moderate pain in 1899. Aspirin is derived from salicylic acid, which had been used for decades to treat pain and fever, but which was beset with side effects, especially a tendency to cause stomach ulcers. Chemists thought that a modification that would release salicylic acid after passage through the stomach would have fewer damaging side effects, and dozens of such variants were synthesized and tested. Aspirin has been the most durable survivor of them all.

One can buy the same dose of aspirin as tablets and capsules at costs ranging from a few pennies to a lot more. What is the difference? Aspirin is made from salicylic acid and acetic anhydride. Open a bottle of very cheap aspirin tablets and smell the stuff; the stinging vinegary odor of acetic acid is often unmistakable. The smell means that the drug has not been purified adequately or that it has decomposed on the shelf, and your stomach will be irritated by these impurities. Naturally, the more carefully recrystallized brands are more expensive, but in this instance economizing does not pay. The manufacturers of the better brands want you to know this, and every day prominent actors promote these products on television. You pay for that advertising on top of the cost of purification and preparation of loosely pressed, more readily absorbed forms. Even so, aspirin (acetylsalicylic acid) remains acidic, and no trick of chemistry or advertising can change that. One way to lessen damage to the stomach wall is to coat the pill with some jellylike basic substance such as aluminum hydroxide (alumina). This buffers the acidity of the drug and reduces the likelihood of ulceration.

Doctors have long known that rheumatic heart disease responds well to large doses of aspirin. Small doses have been credited with reducing the incidence and reoccurrence of heart attacks. A newly recognized drawback of aspirin is that it may precipitate a severe disturbance (Reye's syndrome) in a very small proportion of young children. Aspirin is an organic acid. It has no monopoly on relieving rheumatic and arthritic inflammation. More than a hundred other organic acids, among them ibuprophen, indomethacin, and sulindac, act in a similar way. These newer drugs have some advantages over aspirin. Some reduce inflammation better, and some are better for the relief of medium-grade pain. A number are prescription drugs in this country, and ibuprophen is the only one recently allowed to be sold without prescription.

The action of powerful opiumlike analgesics has been attributed to the intervention of the enkephalins, but the antiinflammatory drugs do not work that way. Seventy-two years after the introduction of aspirin, the British pharmacologist John R. Vane observed in

1970 that this drug interferes with the biosynthesis within the body of some of the prostaglandins. These active chemicals were first isolated from the prostate gland's fluids (hence their name) by the Swedish biochemist von Euler in 1935. However, they occur in extremely small quantities and had puzzling chemical properties that delayed research into their functions. Forty years later, when difficulties in studying these substances could be tackled by new techniques, many scientists became interested in their reactions.

There are many natural prostaglandins, and now there are many hundreds of molecular modifications conceived in the laboratory that have diverse biological properties. There is one, PGE 2, that increases the awareness of pain (lowers the pain threshold) and may serve the natural purpose of alerting the body to disturbances of its normal functions. Another prostaglandin promotes coagulation of the blood; another contracts the uterus, and so forth. All of the natural prostaglandins are made in body cells from a long-chain molecule called arachidonic acid by the action of successive enzymes. Like water falling over rocks, the intermediate substances and the final products cascade down from the arachidonic starting material. Aspirin and the other nonsteroidal drugs block one of the enzymes (cyclooxygenase) in this cascade toward inflammation. Without this crucial step, the inflammatory prostaglandin cannot be made, and swelling, heat, and pain are prevented. This is a wonderful example of how research to explain the action of a natural biochemical system can lead to practical results in quite another area. Since it was learned that these drugs block cyclooxygenase, a simple screening method using this enzyme in test tubes avoids the necessity of using animals—an improvement over the previous tests.

Another equally effective type of drug to relieve headaches and other moderate pains is represented by acetaminophen, which works in a different way from the acidic antiinflammatory medicines. Many patients who fear the effects of acidic preparations on the stomach prefer acetaminophen, which is the active ingredient of most of the "aspirin-free" nonprescription painkillers. The available brands are distinguished by pill size, enteric coating of tablets to prevent their solution in the stomach, and beautiful colors—which, of course, do not contribute anything to dull the pain. The only thing that such beauty treatments assure is a steep increase in price.

Aspirin, acetaminophen, and the other nonsteroidal antiinflammatory analgesics relieve only minor types of pain. Neither type of drug cures the causes of pain, and both give only temporary relief of symptoms, yet the volume of their sales is extraordinary. Figures of eight hundred million dollars per year may be low estimates.

Superficial or surface pain from neuralgias is believed to be helped by local application of oil of wintergreen and similar linaments. Counterirritants can also make one forget such pain for a short time. The pain of itching and skin allergies can be eased by applying hydrocortisone and other steroids to the inflamed area.

The steroid drugs have lost some of their popularity because of their side effects. Cortisone and hydrocortisone (cortisol) are hormones that were isolated from the adrenal cortex over forty years ago and have been synthesized commercially, but their antiinflammatory action cannot be separated satisfactorily from their many different and interdependent biological activities. At first nobody wanted to alter their chemical structure because of the prevalent belief that "Nature knows best," so what chance would a mere chemist have to compete synthetically with chemicals selected by evolution over the eons? However, as in the case of many other natural products, this idea became untenable when Fried and Sabo made changes in some hormones and succeeded in preparing variants much stronger and somewhat more specific than cortisone and cortisol. Since then, hundreds of such analogs have been tested, and as usual, a few survived the demands of clinical trials. To cite just three examples, prednisone, prednisolone, and dexamethasone are widely prescribed steroids for severe cases of rheumatoid arthritis and other inflammatory conditions.

7

Hormones and Vitamins

SEX HORMONES

Extremely small amounts of sex hormones were isolated from the testes, from pregnancy urine, and from the corpus luteum ("yellow body," an endocrine gland that secretes progesterone) and ovaries around 1930. The chemistry of these compounds was studied and brought Nobel Prizes to a string of organic chemists. All of these hormones are steroid derivatives produced from cholesterol in the sex glands and auxiliary glands. The principal female hormone, called estradiol, is broken down (metabolized) by oxidation, and its oxidation products such as estrone are excreted in the urine. Chemists had to process 40,000 liters of urine from pregnant mares to isolate a very few milligrams of estrone. Estradiol and estrone make female animals go into heat (estrus). In women, the estrogens induce the menstrual cycle and ovulation.

The other type of female hormone is progesterone. Its source is the corpus luteum; its mission is to prepare the uterus to receive and embed the fertilized egg (ovum) and to maintain pregnancy to term.

The male sex hormone, testosterone, is needed for the maturation of the male sex organs, for the production of sperm, and for the maturation of secondary male characteristics. Of these, change of voice and growth of beard and body hair are called androgenic effects, while development of male muscles is called the anabolic effect. Muscle development can be increased and separated from sex hormonal activity by some synthetic derivatives of testosterone. These anabolic steroids are taken by mouth by some athletes to build up muscle mass, but this may involve severe health dangers.

Cancers increased by sex hormones can be treated with the opposite sex hormone. Cancer of the breast is retarded by androgens, and prostatic cancer by estrogens. Molecular modification of the natural hormones has produced variants with more specific effects that are preferred for treating specific problems. Totally synthetic estrogens have also been made; the synthetic diethylstilbestrol has advantages over estradiol—it is cheaper and can be used in veterinary medicine for farm animals. However, it has been accused of causing cancer. An analog of diethylstilbestrol called tamoxifen is used in breast cancer of premenopausal women.

The greatest success of molecular modification in this area has come from synthesizing analogs of progesterone. The natural hormone must be injected because it is not active when taken by mouth. A synthetic variant with two slight changes in the original progesterone structure is active as a pill and can be used by women to imitate the conditions of pregnancy, in which fertilization cannot take place. That means that a sexually active woman is protected from becoming pregnant. This is the principle underlying the contraceptive pill. To approximate the conditions of monthly hormonal changes and keep a woman on her usual non-pregnant, chemical course, a weak estrogen (such as estrone methyl ether) is incorporated in "the Pill." The changes in population control and in the sexual liberation of millions of women brought about by these drugs need no further comment.

INSULIN

Insulin is a hormone secreted by the beta cells of a tissue in the pancreas. Its function is to regulate the level of blood sugar (glucose). Lowering the normal amount of glucose leads to hypoglycemia. Because all organs, especially the brain, depend on glucose for energy, too little blood sugar will interfere with normal energy-requiring activities. When glucose levels are raised—as after a meal—high blood sugar (hyperglycemia) results. In normal individuals, glucose returns to average concentrations (100 mg in 100 ml of blood) quite rapidly, but if something goes wrong with the supply of insulin, glucose levels remain high and the extra glucose will be excreted in the urine. This happens in diabetes.

Insulin keeps the level of blood sugar normal in several ways. One is its effect on the passage of glucose molecules through the membranes that enclose tissues. Ordinarily glucose can cross tissue membranes easily. It is stored in the tissue cells after being polymerized into a starchlike material called glycogen. This storage process removes glucose from the circulation. Part of the circulating glucose is also oxidized or burnt up with the catalytic help of insulin, which again lowers the levels of blood sugar. If there is not enough insulin, too much glucose remains in the blood.

Insulin is a medium-sized protein with an amino acid composition that differs slightly in different animals. In spite of their molecular complexity, artificial insulins have been synthesized in England, China, and the U.S.A. Many related proteins have also been made in the laboratory. One of the practical aims of these experiments has been to prepare a hormonelike protein that can be taken by mouth instead of having to be injected, but so far this goal has not been reached.

Diabetic patients, especially those who have suffered from diabetes since childhood, have to replenish their inadequate insulin by injecting commercial insulin daily. Obviously insulin cannot be taken from human glands; therefore, animal pancreas glands (beef, pork, sheep) are extracted instead. Unfortunately, there are occasional allergic reactions to animal insulins, but human insulin has not come on the market until very recently. This new supply is a triumph of genetic engineering by scientists applying the recombinant DNA technique. Specially treated yeast or bacterial cells *(Escherichia coli)* are exposed to human pancreatic beta cells and adopt their genes (portions of nucleic acids) that make insulin. These genes, when incorporated into the bacterial genetic machinery, make the bacteria behave, in part, like the human cells. From then on, they make large quantities of human insulin, which can be purified and used to replace the scanty hormone in patients.

In an unrelated series of events, French chemists noticed that treating animal infections with some of the sulfa drugs (sulfanilamides) lowered the levels of their blood sugar. By systematically changing the structure of these antibacterial drugs, German chemists developed compounds that were no longer antibacterial but had become antidiabetic. These sulfonylurea drugs can be taken by mouth; they improve the kind of diabetes that begins at an advanced age but are ineffective against juvenile diabetes. Like so many other drugs, the sulfonylureas have some undesirable side effects, but their clinical advantages generally outweigh these drawbacks.

OTHER HORMONES

The hormones of the thyroid gland are relatively simple amino acids containing iodine. The two most active of these are thyroxine and triiodothyronine. They are made by the gland from iodide salts in the diet. People who live where iodine in soil and water is scarce do not get enough in their food and suffer from goiter and other deficiency diseases, which today are largely prevented by the addition of iodide to table salt. Medical knowledge of thyroid hormones has advanced to the point where their production, action, and receptors are understood. Among other activities, these hormones help to control the rate at which the body uses energy. People with too few thyroid hormones are sluggish, while those with too many are overactive.

Hormones of the pituitary gland and other brain components are small peptides (proteinlike substances). They are composed of amino acids arranged either in lines or in rings. Very small differences in these arrangements make a lot of difference in their activities. These structural variations suggest that the hormones evolved in different ways to meet the individual needs of various kinds of animals.

Several of these small hormones have been synthesized. By incorporating radioactive atoms into their amino acids, such as ^{14}carbon instead of the usual ^{12}carbon, it is possible to follow the path of a hormone through the body. The blood carries it to the tissues containing its receptors. If these tissues are laid over an X-ray film, the radioactive hormones will leave black spots on the film, thus pinpointing the exact location of their action. Included in the things that the pituitary hormones do are the contraction of the uterus, changing the blood pressure, regulating calcium metabolism, and stimulating certain glands to secrete other hormones.

The growth hormone, also a peptide, can now be used to help the long bones of unusually short children grow more normally. Growth hormone, exceedingly difficult to obtain (from cadavers) until a few years ago, has now become available by recombinant DNA techniques. In the U.S.A., 7,000 to 8,000 children can now have their growth-hormone deficiency (dwarfism) corrected.

The hormones of the adrenal gland have been mentioned before. Lately, nerve cells and endings have been recognized as sources of neurohormones, not unlike glandular tissues in that respect.

VITAMINS

Vitamins are compounds that are needed, usually in small quantities, for numerous metabolic processes in the animal body. If not enough of a vitamin is present in the diet, serious deficiency diseases may result. Like the hormones, vitamins are catalysts, but there is a difference; hormones are made by the body, whereas vitamins have to come from outside, either from the diet or, in some cases, from beneficial microbes that inhabit the body.

Some animals can make certain substances that are vitamins for humans. In such animals these vitamins behave like hormones. For example, the guinea pig like man, cannot produce vitamin C (ascorbic acid), but the rabbit can. Vitamin C is therefore a hormone in the rabbit.

Most of the vitamins are obtained from a normal mixed diet that includes meat, cereals, vegetables, fruit, dairy products, and inorganic salts. An ordinary diet in this country will furnish adequate amounts of vitamins, but in certain cases, when food is not assimilated normally or during stressful periods such as pregnancy, vitamin supplements may be required.

The vegetable kingdom is the principle source of vitamins in our nutrition. The K vitamins come from some vegetable sources but also from intestinal bacteria that synthesize them, and their hosts can then absorb them through the intestinal wall. Vitamin B_{12} comes from liver, Vitamin E from wheat-germ oil, etc.

Almost all of the vitamins have been synthesized, and many are produced commercially. The synthetic vitamins are absolutely identical to the natural vitamins, but of course they are separate chemicals and not mixtures of various compounds, as may be encountered in natural sources. For example, synthetic vitamin E is alpha-tocopherol, while wheat germ oil contains a mixture of tocopherols, not all of which have vitamin activity. The B vitamins often occur together in foods, whereas individual B vitamins are usually synthetic and have to be mixed for complete vitamin B therapy. Commonly the pills contain the required daily minimum dose of each vitamin. For special deficiencies, some more easily metabolized forms of certain vitamins are offered in extra-strength capsules.

Two B vitamins (riboflavin, or B_2, and cobalamine, or B_{12}) are synthesized by molds of the Streptomyces family. The molds are supplied with nutrients that are precursors of the vitamins, and the molds ferment these nutrients to the desired end product. This fermenting process has greatly reduced the cost of these vitamins. Today tons of them are used to enrich foods. Vitamin C is manufactured by a multi-step synthesis in an automated chemical plant with computerized controls and robots, and is supervised by a minimum of human operators.

The vitamins were named by letters in the sequence of their discovery from 1910 to 1950. As their chemistry unfolded, more explanatory generic names were given; thiamine for B_1, riboflavin for B_2, pyridoxal for B_6, etc.

Studies of the structures of the vitamins and their synthesis have been featured highlights of chemistry and rewarded by numerous

Nobel Prizes. The understanding of vitamins and their uses as medicines and for food enrichment have all but eliminated in this country such diseases as scurvy from lack of ascorbic acid, polyneuritis (beriberi) from absence of thiamine, pellagra from too little niacinamide and riboflavin, pernicious anemia from scarcity of cobalamin plus an enzyme called internal factor, rickets from shortage of the D vitamins, and xerophthalmia from want of retinal.

Many other, less drastic deficiencies are helped by vitamin therapy. Considerable debate has surrounded claims that vitamin C prevents or cures colds and allergies. If these claims had not been supported by two eminent scientists, Linus Pauling and Albert Szent-Györgi, they would have been derided by the medical profession. Ascorbic acid is a reducing agent; when taken in huge doses, hundreds of times the established amount needed for ordinary living, it reduces many oxidized compounds, including some that are known to cause cancer, and thereby should lessen their damaging effects. Although the evidence for this explanation is circumstantial, benefits from large doses of the vitamin cannot be denied. Excess ascorbic acid is excreted unchanged, and it appears to be nontoxic. This is not the case for large doses of the A and D vitamins. They disturb the metabolism of minerals. Some claim that vitamin E and a precursor of vitamin A, beta-carotene, retard the development of malignant tumors, but animal tests suggest that large amounts of these substances are risky.

8

Local Anesthetics, Antispasmodics, and Antihistamines

Local anesthetics are used to block the transmission of pain messages to the brain without producing unconsciousness, as in general anesthesia. These drugs perform well when injected into the gum in dental surgery, into muscles and under the skin for minor surgery, or dropped into the eye to avert pain there. They can also be injected into various sections of the spinal cord, where they block the awareness of pain sensations coming from whole sections of the body. A few local anesthetics perform well through the skin and on the lining of the nose and mouth (mucous membranes). These drugs counteract itching and other surface pain. Dentists use them to numb the surface of the gum to avoid pain from later, deeper injections.

For ages people have rubbed all kinds of leaves, oils, and other materials on themselves to blunt topical pain, but numbing underlying tissues was first achieved with cocaine. The dangers of cocaine prompted medicinal chemists to search for other local anesthetics. They thought it likely that the molecular structure of cocaine determined its anesthetic activity, and this idea guided the planning of their research. Piece by piece they chipped away sections from the cocaine molecule until they found structures with local anesthetic activity. Among them were benzocaine and procaine. For a while, procaine became the most widely used injectable local anesthetic, best known by its proprietary name, Novocaine. Benzocaine was even simpler; it has survived for eight decades and is still used on surface tissues.

The success of these drugs, especially procaine, opened floodgates of imitation. Hundreds of similar local anesthetics were made, tested, used, and forgotten over the years. By silent consent, their names all ended in -caine. The French chemist Fourneau translated his name into English (furnace or stove) and named his variety of local anesthetic in his own honor, stovocaine. Most of these drugs had the same drawback: they did not last long enough in the tissues and had to be renewed by a drip technique. Their disappearance is caused by a part of the molecule called an ester group. Ester groups are decomposed by esterase enzymes. Therefore, the chemists explored other, less easily destroyed variants having ether and amide groups. One of these proved to be a long-lasting surface anesthetic, and another, lidocaine (Xylocaine), remains the most widely used, long-lasting, injectable local anesthetic. It was devised by the Swedish chemist Löfgren.

We now know that anesthetics act by blocking microscopic channels through which mineral ions (sodium, potassium, calcium) pass to the interior of nerve cells. The first step in the complicated sequence leading to this blocking appears to be a chemical interference with the nervous transmission of impulses at specific places (nodes of Ranvier) on parasympathetic nerves. Other drugs, such as antispasmodics, block pain messages through the parasympathetic nerves at other locations.

ANTISPASMODICS AND ANTIHISTAMINES

Antispasmodics block the neurohormones, acetylcholine, and sometimes 5-hydroxytryptamine (5-HT, serotonin) from transmitting nervous impulses. They keep muscles from becoming spastic and glands from excessive secretion. Among other actions, they relax the muscles that contract the stomach and intestines. Chemically they resemble biogenic amines, but at one end of their molecules they have one or two bulky, inert structures that act as blocking groups. When, for example, acetylcholine is attracted to receptors, if an antispasmodic is present, the neurohormone will be blocked physically from joining its receptor. On a molecular basis this is very similar to what happens when a football player running for a goal meets two big opponents who block his way and pull him down.

A large number of antispasmodics are available to physicians, led by the ancient alkaloid atropine, which is still one of the most powerful drugs of this type (anticholinergic). When given before an operation, it dries up glandular secretions and relaxes involuntary muscles.

In a similar type of interference, the action of histamine at its receptors (called H-1) is blocked by antihistamines or, as they are now called, H-1 receptor antagonists. These drugs prevent histamine from linking to its receptors by blocking structures similar to those of the bulky antispasmodics. It is easy to understand why drug activities overlap. For example, the antihistaminic drug diphenhydramine not only efficiently counteracts histamine-caused allergic reactions such as running nose and hay fever, but controls muscular spasms as well and even sedates the central nervous system and induces sleep. In fact, many over-the-counter drugs owe their sleep action to diphenhydramine. By slowing down nervous transmission in the cochlear region of the inner ear, the same drug counteracts motion sickness. Travelers can take Dramamine, which is a different salt of diphenhydramine, to prevent sea or air sickness.

Approximately thirty antihistaminic drugs are available for medical treatment. Most of them cause drowsiness and should be avoided by people who must drive an automobile or run machinery. But not all people are sedated by the same agent. Some show no sign of sedation when taking the same drug that puts others soundly to sleep. Physicians and patients must experiment to find out which drug a given patient will tolerate best.

Histamine has another activity that does not respond at all to the typical antihistamine; that is its ability to increase the secretion of hydrochloric acid by the mast cells of the stomach. In certain individuals who are under stress or are genetically disposed that way, stomach acidity will increase enough to cause gastric and duodenal ulcers. Only ten years ago British chemical researchers discovered substances that block this damaging rise in acid. Such drugs are known as H-2 receptor antagonists, and the two most common are cimetidine and ranitidine. They no longer carry the blocking groups that hinder histamine from joining its H-1 receptors. Instead, they are clever variations of the structure of histamine itself. Their chemistry enables them to fasten so tightly to the H-2 receptors that histamine cannot dislodge them to become active.

9

Drugs That Act on the Blood Pressure and the Heart

It is now possible to control both low and high blood pressure with drugs that bring pressure levels in line with more normal measurements. However, these medicines do not cure the causes of abnormal blood pressure. Low blood pressure (hypotension) occurs during periods of starvation, exposure to cold, loss of blood, and surgery. If these difficulties are temporary, it may not be necessary to resort to drugs, but if they persist, a drug to increase blood pressure may be in order. In extreme cases of low blood pressure, epinephrine or its synthetic analog, isoproterenol, which constrict blood vessels, can be tried. Milder cases respond to amphetamine, ephedrine, and similar drugs.

The more serious and insidious change in blood pressure is hypertension. There are many causes of high blood pressure, and no one type of drug will regulate it for everyone. Only a few of the types of hypertension that can now be treated will be discussed here. Some cases are caused by the constriction of blood vessels in the periphery of the body, others by the failure of kidney enzymes that regulate excretion of sodium. Still others are caused by changes in the regulating mechanisms in the central nervous system. A threatening form of high blood pressure is called essential hypertension—a strange name that seems to say that everyone needs it, whereas the opposite is true. Not all of its causes are understood. Persistently high levels of blood pressure overwork the heart and endanger the blood vessels, including those of the brain, and contribute to heart attacks and to "cerebral accidents," which most people call strokes.

Epinephrine (adrenaline) increases blood pressure by narrowing small blood vessels and building up pressure behind these constrictions. As long as this goes on in a normal way, all is well. The action of epinephrine must not be allowed to get out of hand, however. Epinephrine acts on two kinds of receptors, called alpha and beta adrenergic receptors by the late Professor Ahlquist of the University of Georgia. Each of these types has been subdivided (α_1, α_2, β_1, β_2, etc.), on the basis of their location in different parts of the body (heart, lung, brain, etc.). Junction of epinephrine with the alpha receptors increases the force with which the heart contracts and thereby increases the blood pressure. Isoproterenol reacts at beta receptors and can revive a failing heart. Irregular heartbeats, called cardiac fibrillation, can be brought back to a normal rhythm by blocking the beta receptors.

The development of beta blockers (technically called adrenergic beta receptor antagonists) was planned and perfected by Sir J. W. Black in Britain in 1962. Over 400 analogs were tried, and finally propranolol was chosen to control irregularities of the heartbeat. Later on, scientists learned that propranolol also lowered high blood pressure effectively by acting on peripheral nerves and in the brain. Still later, it was observed that this drug reduces pressure in the eye from glaucoma.

Propranolol's interesting health benefits and high sales figures set competitive research in motion in many large pharmaceutical companies. Two of the resulting drugs are nadolol, which is not broken down to any extent in the body but is excreted slowly and therefore acts for a long time, and timolol, which is specific for the treatment of glaucoma. Nadolol can also prevent migraine headaches.

A similar late recognition of pressure reduction occured in the history of thiazide diuretics that were originally designed to treat edema by improving the excretion of water and salt by the kidney. The thiazides are often used in combination with other pressure reducers such as beta blockers.

Epinephrine is the acknowledged cause of some forms of high blood pressure, and it was only natural for chemists to try to block its synthesis in the body. One drug resulting from these efforts is methyldopa, which lowers the blood pressure in some cases by interfering with some of the enzyme catalysts needed to make epinephrine.

Ondetti succeeded in developing a drug that influences kidney enzymes thought to play a role in essential hypertension. After hundreds of attempts he produced captopril, which was patterned on a viper poison that causes a fall in blood pressure. The explanation of the action of captopril and related substances has taxed the imagination of biochemists, who succeeded in unraveling its complicated effects on kidney enzymes.

Every other nerve path involved in changes in blood pressure has been studied, and drugs designed to act at these locations have been tried. Nerve cells cluster around nerve ganglia, which serve as a sort of telephone exchange, and ganglionic blocking agents have been made, tested, and often abandoned. Reserpine still has restricted uses in treating high blood pressure. One reasonable suggestion—to relieve the blood pressure built up behind narrow blood vessels with drugs to dilate the vessels—has had only a limited success.

This short selection of medicines to control high blood pressure is intended to give the reader an idea of the variety of approaches, the groping for rational treatments, and a few selected accomplishments in this difficult and incomplete area of medicinal research.

DRUGS FOR HEART DISEASES

The heart muscle contracts and relaxes rhythmically under the influence of a number of biochemical reactions. Its rhythm is controlled by involuntary (autonomic) nervous impulses. The reactions that power the contractions are mostly exchanges of ions: that is, electrically charged fragments of molecules and atoms. Among them are sodium, potassium, and calcium ions, which flow across cell membranes or, at times, have to be made to flow across. The chemicals that do the transporting are ATP (adenosine triphosphate) and its chemical relatives. Their reactions release energy both as heat and as electricity. This energy is used to convey ions across membranes. Once across, the ions activate proteins in the heart muscle, which then gather together into bundles of fibers. These, in turn, contract and then relax, returning to a resting position. This process is much more complicated than the outline given in these few words. Drugs that stimulate the force of the contractions are called positive inotropic agents (*ino* means muscle and *tropic* means to influence in Greek).

The classical inotropic drugs are the glycosides of digitalis. Dried and powdered, the purple foxglove plant, used since the thirteenth century, was often toxic. In 1785, William Withering showed the inotropic value of digitalis and, by standardizing plant samples and adjusting doses to each patient's needs, recommended ways to reduce its danger. Standardization proved too much trouble for most physicians, and it took another 150 years before digitalis became the accepted medication for hearts that did not contract forcefully enough.

Most physicians prefer to prescribe a purified, well-standardized drug that is now obtained from the wooly foxglove *(Digitalis lanata)* and is called digoxin (Lanoxin). After patients have taken higher doses to establish adequate levels in their blood, they can be maintained on low daily doses.

The contraction of the four heart chambers must not only occur forcefully but also with great regularity in a rhythmic fashion. This process requires the coordination of a complicated system of electric discharges—a pacemaker that regulates the automatic cooperation between the chambers. The two atria at the top of the heart must contract and empty their contents before contraction of the ventricles at the bottom begins. If any of the four fail, the rhythm is broken. Atrial irregularities (arrhythmias) are not regarded with the same dread as ventricular fluttering (fibrillation), which occurs when sections of the lower muscles die after the arteries that supply them with blood have become clogged. Drugs that prevent irregular contractions are called antiarrhythmics. More than half a dozen of these drugs are in use today. Among them is quinidine, an alkaloid occurring in cinchona bark together with its close relative, the antimalarial drug quinine. Unfortunately, quinidine is not well tolerated by a number of heart patients. Like other nonspecific antiarrhythmic drugs, quinidine stabilizes the membranes of heart cells by checking the flow of certain ions through them, reducing their permeability.

Other nonspecific drugs apparently work the same way and help some patients by stabilizing irregular beats. Two of these are local anesthetics, lidocaine and procainamide, and are used widely during heart attacks. Phenytoin, designed to control convulsions, also stops fibrillation. In all these cases, the action on the heart was discovered after the drug had been introduced for other uses.

Propranolol and a number of related drugs were designed to control heart rhythms, tested for that purpose, and introduced into cardiology as useful tools. Their usefulness in other ways, such as lowering high blood pressure and preventing painful attacks of angina pectoris, was discovered later. On the other hand, the drug verapamil was tested for relief of angina during its development and studied with special attention to its action on the flow of calcium ions through heart cell membranes.

The first effective drug to relieve anginal pain was the liquid amyl nitrite, available since 1867. Some more stable nitrogen compounds have replaced amyl nitrite, especially nitroglycerin (glycerol trinitrate). This high explosive, the active component of dynamite, had opened the era of modern blasting and earned the Swedish mining engineer Alfred Nobel the fortune that still finances the Nobel Prizes. The bother of having to place capsules of nitroglycerin under the tongue and await the action of the drug has fueled research for substances that could be swallowed. The new drugs mannitol and isosorbide nitrate, and nitrate esters of several other carbohydrates, fulfill this requirement but are still slow to act.

DIURETICS

Diuretics not only increase urine flow but help the excretion of excess salts and ions by triggering their selective filtration in the kidney.

The fluids of the mammalian body are very similar to seawater, from which all animals arose. Their concentration of salts, especially ordinary salt (sodium chloride), is one-fourth that of seawater: namely, about 0.23 percent. This holds for blood, lymph, tears, saliva, stomach fluid, etc. Solutions with equal salt content are called isotonic. Some body fluids are acidic (stomach juice); some are alkaline (intestinal juice, saliva); others, like blood serum, are neutral.

Blood circulates through all body organs including the kidney, which contains yards of fine tubes coiled inside. In the kidney the blood is separated into its components by a complicated process of absorption and filtration. Each kidney cell (nephron) lets water and electrically charged atomic particles (electrolytes) pass into the tubules while returning blood corpuscles and nutrient molecules to the circulation. Not all charged particles are allowed to pass through the kidney tubules. This selective filtration keeps enough electrolytes in the blood to maintain its normal isotonic concentration. If the blood contains too much blood sugar for extended periods, the excess glucose will pass through the kidney and appear in the urine. Proteins do not pass through kidney membranes unless the kidney is infected or otherwise damaged. The appearance of protein in a cloudy urine is a sign of kidney disease.

Salts must be dissolved in about 99 percent of water to stay at isotonic concentration. If excess ions—of sodium, for instance—are to be filtered out and discarded in the urine, corresponding amounts of water must accompany them. Likewise, if excess ions accumulate in the body, its tissues will swell because of the water that holds the salts. This condition is called edema and occurs during kidney diseases, toxemia of pregnancy, premenstrual tension, and as a side effect when steroids are taken for a long time. The most common cause of edema is congestive heart failure, in which the heart cannot pump blood through the kidney well enough to allow the kidney to filter properly.

Stirring the kidney to greater activity (diuresis) can be done by many chemicals. Several of them are only historically interesting; drugs containing mercury, such as mercaptomerin and meralluride, are still used occasionally. Caffeine found in coffee, tea, and cola drinks is mildly diuretic but is not used clinically. It belongs to a class of chemicals called xanthines, of which theophylline is more effective as a diuretic. Theophylline is usually combined with other, more active substances.

The drug triamterene can let sodium be filtered out into the urine while leaving potassium behind. Usually these two ions go or stay together. In combination with the more powerful sodium-excreting drugs, triamterene has filled an important place among kidney drugs.

Probably the most widely used diuretics stem from the thiazides; chlorothiazide and hydrochlorothiazide were the first to be prescribed. In addition to being diuretics, they lower the blood pressure, a valuable aid in congestive heart failure. The thiazide studies followed the discovery that certain sulfa drugs (sulfanilamides) block an enzyme (carbonic anhydrase) that, in the kidney, changes the acidity of the urine. Blocking this reaction increases the flow of urine. The first successful diuretic that blocked this enzyme was acetazolamide, synthesized and tested by Richard O. Roblin, Jr. The drug also blocks the same enzyme in other organs, e.g., in the eye, where it reduces the pressure from glaucoma. The thiazides are clever chemical relatives of the carbonic anhydrase blockers but act by a variety of different mechanisms. They were first developed by the industrial scientists James M. Sprague, F. C. Novello, and K. H. Beyer.

Thousands of sulfa compounds were tried, and furosemide was found in the Hoechst Laboratories in Germany. It is a high-ceiling diuretic, i.e., it acts by inhibiting sodium and chloride transport in the ascending loop of Henle in the kidney. Ethacrynic acid increases the flow of urine by acting on kidney filtration as a loop diuretic.

Blocking any hormone that tends to retain fluid in the body would seem to be a logical idea to increase the flow of urine, but this is easier said than done. In the case of aldosterone (an antidiuretic hormone made in the adrenal cortex), these efforts produced the drug spironolactone, which bars aldosterone from its receptors.

There are several less important diuretics, and research to discover others with a different type of action goes on all over the world. So far this work has given physicians a variety of drugs for relieving hypertension, edema, kidney failure, and congestive heart failure.

10

Intestinal Tract Medications

The most objectionable feature of commercial television broadcasts is their bad taste in advertising, and of these advertisements the discussion of laxatives is the worst. The bathroom should be a private place, but the networks disagree with this opinion. If laxatives must be aired for commercial reasons, the public should be spared the knowing wink of the actors on the TV screen and insinuations that these drugs are important new discoveries. In fact, most of them have been around for a long time.

Several classes of drugs affect the stomach and intestinal tract, but only three types will be discussed: the cathartics, the constipating drugs, and the antacids. If one is to believe the TV commercials, antacids and laxatives greatly interest many people, so they come first.

Stomach antacids lower the acidity of the stomach (gastric) contents. Too much acid (hyperacidity) is evident in heartburn or hiatal hernia in which a break in the diaphragm that divides the upper chest from the stomach allows some fluids from the stomach to pass back up instead of all moving downward. Acidity is also apparent in inflammation of the stomach or pancreas, in gallstone problems, and in cases of angina pectoris. The excess stomach acid (hydrogen chloride) can be neutralized with baking powder (sodium bicarbonate) or with calcium carbonate, which goes into solution more slowly. Milk of magnesia (8 percent magnesium hydroxide) and other magnesium compounds form the active ingredients of the many tablets that executives take on television when the company's profits are down. All these basic salts (hydroxides, silicates, and phosphates) neutralize some of the stomach acid. Aluminum hydroxide is gelatinous and coats the stomach lining, protecting it for a while from the overly acid stomach juices.

None of these neutralizers remove the cause of surplus acidity. Stress, excessive secretion of histamine, and spastic reactions of the muscles of the stomach and intestine are at the bottom of the condition and may, in extreme cases, lead to ulcers. Drugs that go to the physiological root of the problem and come close to being curative are cimetidine and ranetidine (histamine-2 receptor blockers).

One of the causes of constipation (intestinal atony) is loss of the successive, involuntary movements of the intestinal muscles, called peristalsis. Stress, faulty diets, dehydration, and prolonged use of constipating drugs may lead to peristaltic slowdown. Many people suffering from constipation reach for over-the-counter laxatives (from Latin *laxare*, "to loosen"), or cathartics (from Greek *kathartikein*, "to purify"). They irritate the intestinal wall and thereby increase its movements. Some of them are inorganic salts such as sodium sulfate; epsom salt (magnesium sulfate), the favorite cathartic of our grandmothers; and milk of magnesia. Others are organic compounds; some of these were found originally in herbs, and others are purely synthetic.

The most widely advertised laxative is phenolphthalein. It has been known as an acid-base indicator since 1880. In acids it is colorless; in bases it is red, a trait useful for adjusting solutions to neutrality. The chemist von Vamossy used phenolphthalein as an indicator of the acidity of cheap wines, as required by the Hungarian government in 1900, and found that it was not toxic and had no effect on dogs. In humans, however, it caused soft stools. Extended studies led to its introduction as a relatively harmless cathartic. It is tasteless itself but is sometimes coated with chocolate; it damages no vital organs; and it activates the muscles that move the large bowel. The commercial potential of this substance as a cathartic has stimulated the development of many similar substances. One of them, acetophenolisatin, is said to be a stronger cathartic than phenolphthalein.

Among botanical cathartics widely used in Europe and the East are several anthraglycosides that occur in leaves, roots, and pods of aloe, frangula, rhubarb, senna, and other plants. The properties of some of them or their decoctions were known to ancient Arabs, Africans, West Indian witch doctors, and California Indians. The senna products are produced commercially; they are mild laxatives. Aloe species in Curacao and East and South Africa furnish similar drugs.

The constipating chemicals have the opposite action from that of the cathartics. Loose stools and diarrhea may be caused by infections, by other diseases of the intestines, by overeating, or by cancers, or they may have psychological causes. Overactivity of the colon and other intestinal segments may be toned down by Lomotil (diphenoxylate), a drug found by Janssen in Belgium during a search for a painkiller. The constipating effects of the complex activity of opium, Paregoric, Pantopon, morphine, and codeine are well known. Materials that absorb other chemicals, fill the colon, and make intestinal contents thicker are used by many people because of their lack of side effects. Kaolin, pectin (Kaopectate), and various bismuth salts (Pepto-Bismol) are among these preparations. None of them removes the causes of the intestinal overactivity, but they offer temporary relief from annoying symptoms and malaise. Infections leading to long-term diarrhea must be treated with antibiotics.

11

Drugs for the Treatment of Cancer

Forty years ago there was not one drug to suppress or cure any cancer; thirty years ago there were two, nitrogen mustard and methotrexate. Today, several dozens medicines are available to treat leukemias, some rare cancers, and even some widely found solid tumors. In a very few cases cures have resulted, especially in the rare and virulent choriocarcinoma and in Burkitt's lymphoma. The other chemotherapeutic drugs only slow down the multiplication of malignant cells. If such agents reach circulating cancer cells before they settle down in a tissue, they can retard growth so much that parts of the body's immune mechanism, the scavenger blood cells (phagocytes), can take up and digest the malignant cells and thus cure the incipient disease. This treatment works best when the disease is in its earliest stages. Unfortunately, diagnosis of cancers is seldom made at these stages, and chemotherapy becomes progressively less effective as cancers invade tissues and become better established. To be sure, the situation is not hopeless even in somewhat later stages. Surgery and radiation will remove or destroy cancerous tissue, but at a price; normal neighboring tissue is always affected. Combination of all three treatments, surgery, radiation, and chemotherapy, offers the best current hope of arresting the spread (metastasis) of cancers. It is against this background that anticancer drugs must be measured.

Cancer is not one disease but an estimated group of over one hundred diseases of different organs. For such a variety of diseases there must be a variety of causes: environmental, dietary, and inherited dispositions to faulty metabolism. All these factors lead to one complete start, a permanent change (mutation) in a cell that causes errors in the directions for constructing genes or for making proteins. In the last few years, the genes that can trigger the change from normal to malignant cells have been identified and named oncogenes. Their composition and location on a chromosome has also been established. This long chemical stride forward in pinpointing a cause of cancers will undoubtedly speed the search for ways to stop the oncogenes from beginning their deadly work. The ultimate causes of carcinogenesis remain uncertain. One reasonable suggestion is that the formation of free radicals—that is, unstable parts of molecules—causes a greater reactivity of various body chemicals, especially with oxygen. In this way peroxides are formed, which aggressively attack otherwise sluggish and stable biochemicals. By altering these biochemicals, the peroxides initiate mutations. Evidence for this is seen in the ability of antioxidants to decrease the chances for oxidative reactions. Vitamins C and E, which are established antioxidants, belong to this type of protective chemicals.

There are many external sources that generate free radicals. These include pollutants, cigarette smoke, alcohol, heavy metals (cadmium, lead, etc.), sodium nitrate (a cold-cut preservative), chlorine, aldehydes, sulfur dioxide, ozone, radiation (X rays, overexposure to the sun, cosmic radiation, nuclear by-products, fallout, etc.). Other toxic free radicals can be generated by cooked or rancid foods, mutagens, carcinogens, heated proteins, mold, toxic plant substances, exhaustion, illness, and stress.

Toxic free radicals can damage body proteins and become cross-linked and tangled; tissues can lose their suppleness; arteries can harden; and the susceptibility to cancer can increase.

The common dread of cancer has produced an allotment of large sums of money for research on cancer drugs. Because public funds are allocated by politicians, and since many politicians are elderly, it is not surprising that they should sponsor research that could benefit them as well as their constituents. The slow advances of chemotherapy have shown that money alone cannot buy knowledge. Creative ideas, intuition, and correlation of facts remain the bases of progress in any complex study such as the chemotherapy of tumors.

Moreover, scientists from different fields who are not familiar with each others' methods have to learn to work together. These matters take much time and mental effort.

Only some of the drugs now in wide use to treat human malignancies will be mentioned in this section. However, the reader should be aware that over 250,000 compounds have been tested in animals, mostly mice. Five different mouse tumors are commonly studied. Experience has shown that 95 percent of those compounds that are active against all five mouse tumors are also active against human cancers. Likewise, 95 percent of all drugs effective for human cancers will be effective for the mouse tumors. Only a small number of drugs active in mice have advanced to clinical trials, however, because their greater toxicity in man makes it impossible to try them clinically. Obviously, metabolism differs in humans and mice.

The earliest effective antitumor substances were alkylating agents, and some of them are still in wide use, principally to control leukemias and tumors of the lymph system as well as some virus-caused cancers. They were discovered during World War II.

An Allied supply ship carrying war gas, sulfur mustard, was landing in the harbor of Naples, Italy, to unload its cargo, should the German General Staff, in despair, loosen war gases against American troops. The vessel was bombed, and sulfur mustard spread over the waves. The ship was abandoned, and its occupants were forced into the sea covered with the war gas. Examination of the blood of those that were rescued showed a sharp drop in the number of white blood cells (leucocytes). Alfred Gilman compared this observation with the overabundance of white cells seen in leukemias, but could not apply sulfur mustard to leukemia patients because of its poisonous effects. Mustard gas is an aggressive chemical that reacts with the proteins and nucleic acids of body cells by irreversibly tying their strands together. Chemists soon devised other compounds with the same binding, or "alkylating," quality but with less toxicity. The first were nitrogen mustards, which no longer blistered as the sulfur compounds did. Of the later types, the most successful has been cyclophosphamide. Still, like the earlier drugs, it is not as specific for cancer cells as one would hope, and it also suppresses protective immunological reactions against foreign cells.

Cancer cells, unlike normal body cells, grow in an uncontrolled fashion. They increase to become tissues that push aside surrounding tissues and invade and damage them beyond repair. Often these malignant cells detach themselves from the original "primary" site, swim away in the circulating fluids, and lodge or fasten themselves in remote places, where they continue to multiply. This spreading process is called metastasis. For example, a thyroid cancer cell may metastasize to some internal organ or a limb and become a second thyroid cancer in that distant spot. Of the more than one hundred recognized types of cancer, some grow slowly, others fast, and the fast growers metastasize most vigorously.

Some cancers depend for their multiplication on hormones. Breast cancer is accelerated by estrogens; testicular and prostatic cancer, by male sex hormones. Therefore, surgical removal of the ovaries can retard the growth of breast cancers.

A number of human and animal cancers are attributed to viruses. These infectious particles invade the host cells and force upon those cells their own metabolic mechanisms, especially the manufacture of the viral nucleic acids by which they multiply. In some cases this takeover may lead to continued virus infections; in others to malignant cell growth.

A virus causing leukemia of human T cells (thymus cells) has been identified with the virus that produces acquired immune deficiency syndrome (AIDS). This is a new disease that suppresses immunological control of infections and of certain cancers. No therapy is known to cure AIDS, but a few drugs originally designed as antitumor agents appear to delay some of the symptoms of the disease. Among them are azidothymidine (AZT), an antimetabolite-type agent, and a steroidal antibacterial antibiotic, fusidic acid.

Some medicinal chemists dream of finding a way to block the oncogene portion of a body cell's reproductive machinery so that a virus or some chemical cannot trigger it into causing the change (mutation) leading to uncontrolled cell growth. All genes are segments of nucleic acids—DNA or RNA, which are very long molecules. Some of these nucleic acids are coiled in a double spiral (helix), but they must uncoil to give directions for copying each half when the time comes for a cell to divide, or to give directions for making proteins.

Scientists now know the general pattern of the nucleotide segments, the types of carbohydrates and bases in them, and the nature of the links that fasten the segments together, and they can understand the meaning in one of the segments that will change the directions it gives for making a metabolic substance (metabolite). The new metabolite is likely to act as a metabolite antagonist that interferes with the original substances' production or reactions. Should some chemist modify the oncogene's nucleic acids so as to produce a suitable nucleotide metabolite antagonist, then cancer might be stopped.

However, consider the mathematics of the chances. In each nucleotide segment there can be one of six bases and one of two carbohydrates. If only the hydrogen atoms in them are counted, each carbohydrate has about six and each base has four or five, and there are also two to four nitrogen atoms that can be replaced or shifted around. Add these numbers, and observe that the possible variations would result in tens of millions of potential metabolite antagonists. It might take half a year to make one, and it would take six to eight years to train someone to make them. All told, it would take several generations to cover this ground even if everybody were drafted for the task, not to mention testing the compounds after they were made. Who would be left to raise food or sell automobiles? That is the problem of cancer chemotherapy. For three decades dedicated chemists have synthesized thousands of metabolite substitutes and equally dedicated biologists have tested them. A few are suitable to test in the clinic, but these are just a drop in the bucket to what it would take to find effective drugs against all cancers. It is almost a miracle that any have been found at all.

Some of the new drugs block enzymes that put the segments together to form the long nucleic acids. Others enter into a segment themselves, but do not fit the code and so prevent the nucleic acids from functioning. Examples are two widely used antimetabolites: 6-mercaptopurine made by George Hitchings and 5-fluorouracil synthesized by Charles Heidelberger.

Whether an active drug will be found is always a gamble, and compounds with no relation to known effective substances are not likely to be studied. Nevertheless, some totally unexpected chemicals have turned out to be effective against some cancers. The best known of these are antibiotics. The original antibiotics were organic compounds obtained from fermentation products of microbes, some of which can retard the multiplication of disease-causing microorganisms, parasites, or cancer cells. The first antitumor antibiotics came from the *Actinomyces* molds, and the only useful one is actinomycin D, which is too toxic for most cases. Another group of antibiotics active against several human cancers are the bleomycins, originally fermented by *Streptomyces verticillatus*. Finally, doxorubicin (adriamycin) is obtained by fermentation from *Streptomyces peucetius*. The last two have been synthesized.

These substances bind to DNA and thus prevent it from uncoiling to make the RNA directions for protein synthesis and even to begin cell division.

A completely different substance with anticancer activity is the inorganic compound *cis*-platinum (*cis*-dichlorodiammineplatinum (II)). This agent, never suspected of having biological importance, was tested by Rosenberg in 1967 against intestinal bacteria and later as an antitumor drug. It may act similarly to the alkylating agents. Although it is toxic, its value in cancer treatment is undisputed.

Among the natural alkaloids tested against rodent tumors, those from the periwinkle plant *(Vinca)* are especially useful in childhood leukemias. They are vinblastine and vincristine.

A cancer specialist cannot always determine the biochemical reactions to which the cancer might be most sensitive. Therefore, cancer treatment rests on the practical assumption that multiple attacks by various drugs are more likely to hit the tumor. This is why pharmaceutical firms usually mix three or more drugs in one tablet, capsule, or injectable preparation. The most common combinations are one alkylating agent, one antimetabolite, and one antibiotic (bleomycin or adriamycin), with *cis*-platinum, vincristine, or other substances added as needed, depending on the type of cancer. Such shotgun treatment has produced some cures and raised the five-year rate of remission for some malignancies to 50–75 percent.

DRUGS AFFECTING THE IMMUNE RESPONSE

For centuries, survivors of some diseases, such as smallpox, have been known to be immune to a second infection. The first infection by viruses or other pathogens produces a toxic chemical called an antigen. After ten to twenty days some new proteins are built patterned on the antigen. These new proteins are called antibodies, and they neutralize the effect of any new dose of antigen that may enter the body on a subsequent occasion. The acquired immunity may last for a short while or for a lifetime. Immunization with specially prepared antibodies may thus have to be given only once, as in the case of poliomyelitis, or at regular intervals, as for smallpox, typhoid fever, cholera, yellow fever, influenza, etc. This type of immunity is termed humoral.

The second type of immune response is mediated by cells of the thymus gland (T cells) and the bursa (B cells, perhaps from the bone marrow). These responses cause delayed hypersensitivity, as encountered in allergies, and in some cases protection against infection. The most serious consequence of cell-mediated immune response is rejection of foreign materials such as grafts and organ implants. Suppression of this response could lead to some kind of acceptance of transplanted organs, and resistance against some diseases that produce cells or tissues rejected by the body as if they were foreign to the organism. Of a long list of such diseases, only a few shall be mentioned: psoriasis, myasthenia gravis, multiple sclerosis, rheumatoid arthritis, lupus erythematosus, rheumatic heart disease, and perhaps early-onset diabetes.

One type of cell arising from normal body cells by mutation and then becoming "foreign" to the body is the cancer cell. When cancer chemotherapy became a clinical reality, virtually all anticancer drugs were also tried to supress cell-mediated immune responses. The results have been variable; at best, these drugs did their job for only a limited time and then lost their suppressive activity. Generations of organ-transplant patients and patients with autoimmune diseases have had to contend with this diminishing suppression. Changing the drugs sometimes extends the period of suppression, but only seldom could this suppression be maintained for a prolonged time.

In the case of methotrexate, a typical sequence of events was seen. The drug was active, but only at high doses that caused considerable toxicity. Because methotrexate is a dihydrofolic acid (= vitamin) antagonist, dihydrofolic acid was administered to patients simultaneously. This counteracted the toxicity of methotrexate without completely ruining its anti-immune response effect—at least for some time.

Among the agents tested were all the antitumor agents, including some antibiotics. A virtual revolution in immunosuppressive therapy occurred when one of these antibiotics, cyclosporin A, was tried. This is a peptide consisting of eleven amino acids arranged in a large ring shape. It was discovered by a Swiss research team in 1976 by fermenting the fungi *Cylindrocarpon lucidium* and *Trichoderma polysporum*. Its peculiar molecular composition makes it resistant to gastric digestion, and the drug can be taken orally. It is much more effective in suppressing cell-mediated immune responses than any other agent used previously.

An unexpected application of cyclosporin is in the treatment of early-onset diabetes. It now appears likely that childhood diabetes may be caused by an abnormal genetic tendency of the child's T cells to destroy the beta cells of the pancreatic islets of Langerhans that produce insulin. Administration of cyclosporin to such individuals, even without the customary doses of maintenance insulin, has given favorable results in suppressing the symptoms of the disease.

Coagulants and Anticoagulants

Blood circulates through large, small, and minutely small vessels. Its fluidity is maintained by numerous biocatalysts that keep blood from clotting within the vessels and that keep it from leaking through the vessel walls. Unwanted clotting may lead to thrombosis, while improper leakage results in hemorrhage. Coagulants prevent hemorrhage; anticoagulants prevent thrombosis.

Blood clotting results from several phases, concerned with the formation of prothrombin from plasma proteins that are labeled by Roman numerals. Prothrombin is converted to a short-lived catalyst called thrombin. Under the influence of thrombin, the water-soluble protein fibrinogen is polymerized and forms an insoluble fibrous material called fibrin. Blood corpuscles get enmeshed in fibrin, and this mixture is the blood clot.

This highly simplified representation of the clotting process would suggest that it can be speeded up or interrupted at many stages, and indeed, that is true. Vitamin K—which is present in alfalfa, spinach, cabbage, soybean oil, egg yolk, etc., and is also synthesized by friendly intestinal bacteria—aids some of the early steps of blood clotting. Conversely, persons who lack factor VIII suffer from hemophilia, a serious inheritable bleeding disorder.

There are several K vitamins; one of them with a simple chemical structure is called menadione. It is used to still bleeding in surgery and other traumatic events. There are water- and oil-soluble derivatives of menadione. Vitamin K does not enter into the proteins of blood coagulation but acts as an essential cofactor.

For minor cuts that cause bleeding, astrigents such as alum can be used. More serious bleeding may require a corticosteroid, aminocaproic acid, and other prescription drugs.

Two types of anticoagulants are in clinical use. One is injectable heparin and related products, the other dicumarol and similar substances that can be taken orally. They are used to prolong blood-clotting time in patients whose blood vessels have already been clogged by a clot after a cardiac or cerebral infarct or by clots in other locations.

Heparin is an unusually structured polysaccharide not unlike starch but solubilized by water-related groups. It was discovered by a medical student at Johns-Hopkins University in 1916. It is extracted from beef lung or liver; it has to be injected and cannot be administered otherwise. It inhibits the formation of thrombin from prothrombin and thereby prevents the clotting mechanism.

The need to inject heparin makes it inconvenient to use for patients who have to take an anticoagulant continuously. It was therefore a fortunate circumstance when the orally active anticoagulants of the coumarin type were developed. The path of this discovery is interesting. In 1922 Schofield called attention to a serious disease of cattle in the upper Midwest. The animals suffered from internal bleeding that was traced to their fodder, improperly cured sweet clover hay. Link at the University of Wisconsin isolated the responsible toxic product and later synthesized it. He called it dicumarol. The compound was introduced as a clinical anticoagulant in 1941.

Molecular modification of this substance provided several more or less related anticoagulants. Only two will be mentioned. One is diphenadione, a drug acting like dicumarol by preventing prothrombin biosynthesis. Diphenadione must be given with caution, since hypersensitivity and bleeding may occur. The other oral anticoagulant to be spoken of here is warfarin. It is also used as a rat poison. It causes hemorrhagic death of these animals.

13

Drugs for Infectious Diseases

Everything that lives, metabolizes, and multiplies by some means of reproduction depends on the chemicals in other living or dead cells and tissues for survival. Herbivore animals feed on plants; carnivore animals feed on animal tissues. Snakes devour living rodents; tigers kill their prey before feeding on them. Man takes a middle road, using vegetables, fruit, live animals (marine shell organisms), and dead animals for his diet. Cannibalistic animals such as seabirds kill their own kind before devouring them, but they eat live fish that are still flapping around while being ingested. Cannibalistic humans are still to be found more often than one wants to admit.

Microbes are organisms at the bottom of the plant and animal kingdoms, but their dietary requirements are not much different from those of higher animals or carnivore plants. Microbes need the building blocks of proteins, nucleic acids, many hormones, some vitamins ("growth factors"), fats, and carbohydrates to survive, to reproduce, and to supply the energy for their life processes. Some microbes invade foreign organisms and live with them in cooperative arrangements. Many symbiotic bacteria inhabit the intestinal tract of mammals, feast on the diet of their hosts, and furnish the host in return with essential biocatalysts, such as certain vitamins that the bacteria can synthesize while the host cannot achieve that. Some of these bacteria digest cellulose for the host, converting it to glucose that the host (ruminant animal, termite) can then utilize.

In many other cases a microbial invasion of man or beast will take its toll of the host organism. Infectious organisms not only use the hosts' biochemicals for their own nutrition but usually metabolize them to materials that are toxic to the host animal and, in sufficient amounts, will kill it. In a way, this is shortsighted of Nature's household. After the death of the host animal, the flow of its biochemicals stops, and the invading microbes will die from the lack of needed nutrients.

When people talk about infections, they usually think of the many infectious diseases that befall humans, domestic and farm animals, pets, and wildlife. But infections are also common among other forms of life. Viruslike particles (bacteriophages) assault bacteria; some bacteria dislodge others from their source of nutrition; and so on. An endless chain of predatory events threatens every living cell and even subcellular particles in a steady fight for survival. On the highest level, humans hunt and destroy food animals, and they destroy other humans by warfare. There is no mercy in Nature. If there is any redemption in these ceaseless battles, it is that some microbes can be kept from reproducing by the use of some chemical weapons against them. Such drugs are bacteriostatic, virustatic, etc. If a drug kills the invading microbe, it will be bactericidal, virucidal, and so forth.

A new weapon used in warfare usually takes a heavy toll of the unprepared victim of the attack. After the surprise has worn off, the victim will often find ways to avoid the same kind of attack on future occasions. Likewise, infectious microbes will succumb to a new foreign chemical that inhibits some of the enzyme catalysts essential for their life processes. After a number of these experiences, and with a continued indomitable destiny to survive, microbes will search for means to avoid the inhibition of their vital enzyme systems. Their metabolism will invent reactions that do not need these enzymes. These shortcuts or circumventions are called metabolic shunts. When such shunts become established, the microbe will no longer be affected by attacks on its previously essential enzymes. It will have become resistant to the drug.

All chemotherapeutic drugs have in common a fundamental mechanism of action. They are directed against the life processes of the invasive, pathogenic organism. Drugs will stop, or interfere with, the biosynthesis or utilization of the building blocks of the invader. These can be constituents of the cell membrane or of the cell nucleus of the pathogenic cell. Usually the action of drugs is directed against protein synthesis, be it the biosynthesis of one of the amino acids that make up the proteins, or the assembly of the amino acids into a large protein molecule. Other drugs interrupt the biosynthesis of the constituents of nucleic acids; they can also interfere with the assembly of these pieces into nucleic acids, or with the utilization of the nucleic acids to transmit commands for protein synthesis. All this goes on in the chemotherapy of *all* invading cells or organisms, be they bacteria, viruses, amoebae or other protozoa, fungi, pathogenic yeasts, or malignant tumor cells. Chemotherapy is essentially a strategic blockade, aimed at the slow death or destruction of the cells to be halted. In most cases, the defenses of the animal body, the phagocytic blood cells, will try to overcome the infectious invaders by enclosing and digesting them, but these defense cells cannot overcome the ever increasing number of the attacking pathogens. That is where chemotherapy comes in. Drugs either kill the pathogens or make it impossible for them to reproduce. The body's defense cells then take care of the smaller enemy armies.

CLASSIFICATION OF PATHOGENIC PARASITES

Disease-causing (pathogenic) foreign organisms range from minute bodies without membranes to multicellular animals that invade host animals. Only a few of these will be catalogued here, and only those that cause the more common infectious diseases observed in moderate climatic latitudes. Some of these infectious organisms belong in the plant kingdom, others are the lowest or at least low forms of animal life. Some, such as the viruses, have affinities to plant or animal cells but are neither themselves.

Viruses are the simplest forms of life. They are microscopic assemblies of genetic material, either DNA viruses or RNA viruses. The nucleic acids are encapsuled in protein (a capsid) that sometimes also contains carbohydrate and lipid components. Viruses can infect plants, insects, bacteria, or animals. They depend on the host cells for nutrients and energy. Animal viruses—the most important in medicine—attach themselves to the surface of the host cells and penetrate into the cell. The protein capsid detaches itself from the nucleic acid material, and this bared genetic substance begins to direct the host cell to synthesize the proteins and enzymes needed by the virus. These new substances, manufactured by the subjugated host cell at the command of the invader, are assembled to form a new virus that is then extruded and can now infect a new host cell. The few chemotherapeutic drugs found that are effective in viral diseases interfere at some of these stages of viral life processes.

Of the hundreds of viral diseases, only a few may be mentioned at random: the common cold, poliomyelitis, viral encephalitis, some forms of leukemias and other cancers, herpes, influenza, yellow fever, acute respiratory disease, smallpox, fowl plague, and AIDS.

Bedsoniae and Rickettsiae have rudimentary cell walls and resemble bacteria more than viruses. They can synthesize some proteins, and they live mostly inside host cells. Among diseases caused by Bedsoniae are psittacosis (parrot fever disease) and lymphogranuloma venereum. Rickettsiae are transmitted to man by tick bites and produce such infections as Rocky Mountain spotted fever.

There are several other pathogens that have characteristics between viruses and bacteria. Some of them cause dangerous human diseases. The differences between them are largely their gradual independence from host cells, some more sophisticated nutrient requirements, and thereby their susceptibility to drugs that interfere with some new life processes. Among these organisms is a mycoplasma that causes primary atypical pneumonia ("viral pneumonia"). L-forms, spheroblasts, and protoplasts are extruded by some bacteria or at least revert sometimes to bacterial forms. They have cell walls, although sometimes defective, are resistant to penicillin and similar antibiotics, and contribute to difficulties in subduing some bacterial infections.

The best studied unicellular organisms enclosed in a rigid cell wall are the bacteria. The bacterial cell wall consists of polysaccharides (celluloselike materials) and proteins that have no analogy in animal membranes. That means that chemotherapy can concentrate on attacking processes that build the bacterial cell wall because such interferences cannot damage cell wall synthesis in the host animal.

Bacteria are free-living organisms that can synthesize their metabolites from simple compounds, including inorganic salts, as long as they contain the essential elements of all living matter. Bacteria can thrive independent of host cells, but in some cases their nutritional requirements have to be produced by host organs. There are some bacteria that need an oxidizing environment (aerobic bacteria), while others get along better under nonoxidizing (anaerobic) conditions. Resistant strains of bacteria, the dread of chemotherapists, emerge through mutation but can be induced by drugs that stimulate bacterial cells to learn to synthesize just those enzymes that the drug inhibits. In other words, the bacterial cell learns to defend itself until the drug loses all its therapeutic value.

Bacterial cells belong substantially to low forms of plant life. The lowest forms of animal cells comprise many types that are pathogenic to mammals, including humans. They belong to the zoological classification of the phylum Protozoa (*protos* = first, *zoion* = animal), one-celled animals that cause a variety of lethal diseases.

Amebiasis is due to *Entamoeba histolytica*, a parasitic protozoan species of ameba with a complicated life cycle. Trypanosomiases are diseases caused by unicellular protozoan parasites of the genus *Trypanosoma*. Both man and animals become infected with trypanosomes through the bite of flies, for example, tsetse flies. In Africa, the human infection is called sleeping sickness; in South and Central America, Chagas' disease. It can no longer be presumed that such infections are restricted to tropical areas of the earth. The rapid exchange of travelers as well as of animals (horses, cattle) and the return of military and industrial personnel from countries where such diseases are endemic has exposed the Northern Hemisphere to outbreaks of a number of "tropical" diseases.

This is especially true of malaria. This group of diseases is transmitted by protozoan organisms of the genus *Plasmodium*. The most dangerous species for humans is *Plasmodium falciparum*, but other forms of malaria caused by *P. vivax* (benign tertian malaria), and *P. malariae* (quartan malaria) also cause much damage, particularly through their high relapse rate. This is due to a recycling of the causative plasmodia, which pass through a multistage life cycle. Plasmodia spend a part of their life stages in *Anopheles* mosquitoes; the infected female mosquito injects the earliest life form of plasmodia, the sporozoites, into their human or animal victims when they feed on their blood.

Chemotherapy made inroads into protozoan infections long before bacterial infections yielded to drugs. Viral diseases cannot yet be treated with reliable and satisfactory drugs; their state of chemotherapy is approximately where the chemotherapy of protozoan diseases was seventy years ago.

CHEMOTHERAPY OF BACTERIAL INFECTIONS

There had been hundreds of attempts to protect patients from bacterial infections, but none of the chemicals tried had fulfilled the two cardinal requirements: high efficiency coupled with low enough toxicity. Many of the old agents were efficient but much too toxic. Others that had acceptably low toxicity were not effective against a sufficiently wide variety of bacteria.

True chemotherapeutic drugs for bacterial infections were first conceived and explored by two great pharmacologists, Gerhardt Domagk and Daniel Bovet. The story of their discovery sheds light on inventiveness and motivation in drug research.

Sulfanilamide, the original prototype of these drugs, was prepared by a German graduate student in 1907, just out of chemical curiosity. It was then forgotten. It is a simple organic compound, and generations of premedical undergraduates in this country have reprepared it as a synthetic exercise during their year in the organic chemical laboratory. In the meantime, Paul Ehrlich suggested that dyestuffs that could stain pathogenic microbes selectively on a microscope slide might kill the same microbes without affecting the surrounding host tissue if they could be made selectively toxic for the pathogens. Ehrlich called this visionary concept chemotherapy, a term he coined for this purpose. Inspired by his vision, every dyestuff—ten thousands of them—in the archives of the dyestuff industry was tried against bacterial cultures in glass dishes and test tubes, but to no avail. The dyestuffs did not stop the multiplication ("growth") of the bacteria.

One gets fed up with doing test after test, each the same way, with nothing as a guide. There were a number of dyestuffs on wool fabrics that had proven to be resistant to sunlight and to washing. Wool is an animal fiber, and consists of fibrous proteins in contrast to cotton, which consists of the polysaccharide cellulose. If a dyestuff adheres to a protein fiber, will it not stain other proteins as well—let us say, bacterial cells? These wool dyes were tried out on the bacterial cultures in their glass containers (*in vitro* = "in glass") based on that hunch, but again they did not work.

At this point, Gerhard Domagk suggested that the wool dyestuffs be tried in bacteria-infected mice. After all, chemotherapy was supposed to protect animals from infections or to heal the infection. And now the miracle happened: mice infected with deadly staphylococci were injected with solutions of those azo dyestuffs, and they recovered—not all of them, but most of them. Peculiarly, only those dyestuffs worked that contained a chemical group called sulfonamide, $-SO_2NH_2$. Encouraged by this breakthrough, the least toxic of the sulfonamide dyes was tried in patients with staphylococcus infections. So confident was Domagk that he chose his own daughter, Hildegard, as the first patient for these trials. She recovered, and her father was offered the Nobel Prize in medicine. The registered trade name of the dyestuff was Prontosil. It was marketed all over the world and began to save the lives of patients with heretofore dreaded infections such as hemolytic streptococci, staphylococci, and similar bacteria. In this country, the son of President Roosevelt, Franklin Delano Roosevelt, Jr., was saved by that drug.

Prontosil (also called Prontosil rubrum because of its red color) became a profitable drug for the German Bayer Company, which held the patent rights. To protect their treasured property, they did not publish the chemical structure of the dyestuff, but it did not take long to break that secrecy. Chemists at the Pasteur Institute of Paris did some detective work, scanning the patents of Bayer Company, and ultimately reconstructed the chemistry of Prontosil. They made many similar dyestuffs in this process to support their conclusions.

The pharmacologist Bovet at the Pasteur Institute kept a colony of mice infected with pathogenic cocci and tested the dyestuffs for curative effects. Something strange happened to the dyestuffs; the urine of the mice was colorless, not red or any other dyestuff color. The mice had metabolized the dye to a colorless compound. This was soon identified. It was a simple derivative of sulfanilamide, synthesized by that graduate student twenty eight years earlier. A bottle of commercial sulfanilamide, a white powdery substance, stood on the shelf at the Pasteur Institute. Indeed, it was used every day to make all those dyestuffs. Bovet tested sulfanilamide and saw that this colorless, nondyestuff drug cured the infected mice. One could ask, Did the German company not observe that also? And if they did, did they keep silent about it because sulfanilamide was an old compound and not protected by a patent? All the people involved in the discovery of Prontosil are gone, and one will never know the truth.

The antibacterial potency of sulfanilamide varied in several in vitro experiments. The British biologists Woods and Fildes treated sulfanilamide-sensitive bacteria with various nutrients in glass dishes and noted that without beef broth present, the bacteria were killed by the drug. With the broth, they were kept from multiplying: that is, sulfanilamide was only bacteriostatic. They analyzed the broth and found it contained *para*-aminobenzoic acid (PABA), an essential growth factor for the bacteria. Woods and Fildes had the presence of mind to compare the chemical formulas of sulfanilamide and PABA. These simple formulas are reproduced here because of their obvious similarity: $H_2N—C_6H_4—CO_2H$ = PABA; $H_2N—C_6H_4—$

SO_2NH_2 = sulfanilamide. We have encountered structurally similar compounds with opposite biological actions before. Here, PABA and sulfanilamide were recognized as the first important pair of metabolic antagonists.

The question still remained why the bacteria needed PABA. It was found that a bacterial enzyme helped PABA to be incorporated in the molecule of the B-complex vitamin, folic acid. Reduced folic acid, in turn, is needed for the synthesis of the purine bases present in nucleic acids. The antagonism of sulfanilamide to the incorporation of PABA into dihydrofolic acid thus deprives the bacteria of the materials in their cell nuclei and thereby of life. Some bacteria that cannot use PABA to synthesize dihydrofolic acid will use prefabricated folic acid from the cells of their host. Such bacteria are not affected by sulfanilamide; they are resistant to the drug.

Sulfanilamide itself was really too toxic for extended routine treatment of infections with cocci. The usual procedure of molecular modification created a long line of analogs with appreciably fewer side effects and with greater potency and longer duration of action. The best analogs also avoided a real drawback, namely, crystallization of drug metabolites in the kidney tubules. Among the analogs that have remained of use in chemotherapy are sulfathiazole, sulfadiazine, sulfisoxazole, sulfasuccidine, and several others. Each of them has its own set of advantages. Sulfisoxazole is well suited to reach bacterial pathogens in the kidney and bladder. Sulfasuccidine removes bacteria from the intestines, an action important for bacterial diarrheas and for cleaning up the intestines before intestinal surgery.

Sulfanilamide and its analogs deny PABA access to an enzyme that helps dihydrofolic acid synthesis. Later on, the dihydrofolic acid has to be reduced by another enzyme, dihydrofolate reductase, before it can participate in the construction of materials needed in the bacterial cell nucleus. Several drugs unrelated to sulfanilamides inhibit the enzyme dihydrofolate reductase, and thereby block all the subsequent steps in this long cascade of biochemical events. If the sulfanilamides block one step and the dihydrofolate reductase inhibitors block another step, would a combination of these two types of drugs not be even better? This was tried by George H. Hitchings, and it worked. A combination of trimethoprim (a dihydrofolate reductase inhibitor) and sulfamethoxazole has become one of the most effective antibacterial agents.

Some patients feel it is a nuisance to have to take a drug several times a day or, in extreme cases, to have to be wakened at night so that they will not miss a dose. Several sulfanilamide derivatives have been found that have half-lives (one-half only having been excreted) of 65 hours and even of 150 hours. However, these attractively long-lasting agents have some drawbacks that have not been completely overcome.

A relative of the sulfonamide drugs, called dapsone, has become the most effective agent for the treatment of leprosy. This ancient and feared mycobacterial infection has surfaced in developed as well as underdeveloped regions. Except for a few virtual reservations (leprosaria) in which patients live together, the Northern Hemisphere is free from this slow-onset infection.

The much more prevalent mycobacterial disease worldwide is tuberculosis. This is also an infection with a slow onset but is difficult to treat chemotherapeutically. An estimated 50,000 chemicals had been tried against tuberculosis in laboratory animals. The first drug to show promise was para-aminosalicylic acid (PAS), but PAS is metabolized quickly, and large doses have to be given (orally) to maintain its concentration in the blood. The mycobacteria also have a tendency to become resistant to PAS.

The sulfanilamides are, on the whole, ineffective against tuberculosis, but the weak activity of one of them, sulfathiadiazole, led Domagk to study some related compounds and to single out even some of the synthetic intermediates needed in the preparation of the substances he wanted to test. Some of these intermediates, called thiosemicarbazones, had a modicum of activity, and the best of them was to be made in a larger quantity for further tests. These experiments were carried out in the pharmaceutical industry, where time is precious. It took a long time to get these syntheses going and the chemists felt hard-pressed to supply samples to the biologists for tests, so they gave them every chemical they had, including, again, some intermediates. And one of these scored: it was isoniazid, which rapidly became (1951) the most important antituberculous drug. It was followed later by ethionamide and pyrazinamide, both industrial products of molecular modification.

These vast efforts involving hundreds of medicinal scientists took place about 1950, when some antibiotics had already made their appearance. Streptomycin and dihydrostreptomycin, introduced by Selma Waksman, were the first antibiotics with activity in tuberculosis. They have been largely abandoned because of their toxicity on the auditory nerves. The antibiotic that has been of great benefit in chronic and drug-resistant pulmonary tuberculosis is rifampicin, a semisynthetic derivative of the rifamycin antibiotics fermented by *Streptomyces mediterranei*. Its very difficult chemical and biological study was performed by Sensi in an Italian pharmaceutical firm.

Bacteria and other microbes are grouped in two large classes, gram-positive and gram-negative. This classification is based on their ability to retain a dyestuff stain originated by Christoph Gram. Gram-positive organisms are, on the whole, more easily affected by drugs than gram-negative ones. There are still many gram-negative bacteria for which no workable drug has been developed. This is true even of antibiotics, although modified penicillins, cephalosporins, and other drugs can be used in some gram-negative infections.

ANTIBIOTICS

Antibiotics are chemicals that interfere with the life processes of pathogenic microorganisms, prevent their multiplication by antagonizing their reproduction, and occassionally destroy the pathogens. The term *antibiotic* was coined by Waksman in 1942 to designate antimicrobial substances produced by other microorganisms. This definition is too narrow and is no longer accepted. There are many antimicrobial chemicals for systemic use that are and always have been purely synthetic, for example, the sulfanilamides. Several natural antibiotics obtained by the fermentation of microbes have been synthesized and are now manufactured synthetically. Many plant products exert antibiotic actions indistinguishable from those of classical fermentation antibiotics. And last but not least, several classical antibiotics kill cancer cells and parasitic multicellular animals, such as pathogenic worms, that cannot be called microbes.

The treatment of infections and infestations with what we would now call antibiotics has been known for thousands of years. Ancient Chinese savants treated boils, carbuncles, and other skin infections with moldy soybean decoctions, the mold serving as a source of an antibiotic. Pasteur and Joubert (1877) found that "common bacteria" could kill cultures of anthrax bacilli and act similarly in anthrax-infected guinea pigs. An impure material exuded by *Pseudomonas aeruginosa* proved of some effect in diphtheria as early as 1890. We now know the material contained two substances: an enzyme called pyocyanase and an antibiotic, hemipyocyanine.

The Naming of Antibiotics—Most names of antibiotics reflect the name of the genus of the microorganism from which they are produced. Thus, penicillin comes from *Penicillium*, polymyxin from *Bacillus polymyxa*. Others have been named for the country or place where the original soil sample was collected. Angolamycin derives from Angola, foromacidin from the Roman Forum, miamycin from Miami. Nystatin relates to the New York *Stat*e Board of Health Laboratories; hamycin to *H*industan Antibiotics, Ltd. Wives of the investigators have furnished some names, e.g., doricin and helenin. Supportive and indispensable secretaries have been the source of other names: nancimycin, vernamycin. Even a mother-in-law's name was drafted for this purpose: Seramycin. A girl by the name of Tracey suffered from a bacillary infection that was cultured and provided the source of bacitracin. Rifamycin was named after the motion picture *Rififi*. Suggestions about other pertinent sources of names will be welcomed by the antibiotics-producing industry.

THE PENICILLINS

Penicillin was discovered by the British bacteriologist Alexander Fleming in September 1928. A culture of staphylococci growing on an agar medium became contaminated by a mold that had been carried to it in the laboratory air from some distance. The bacteria growing in the vicinity of the mold disappeared. Fleming identified the mold as *Penicillium notatum* and realized it must have produced an antibiotic substance, which he named penicillin. He showed also that this fermentation product did not make the culture medium toxic to white blood cells and proposed that penicillin might be useful as an antiseptic. The day of systemically active antibacterials had not yet arrived (Prontosil surfaced in 1932), and it never occurred to Fleming to explore any systemic action of penicillin.

The discovery of penicillin casts another sidelight on the working habits of bacteriologists of that day. Eleven years later, after the outbreak of World War II, a young University of Virginia student enlisted in the RAF, since he was itching to get into the fray but the United States was still neutral. After his arrival in England, his commanding officers had second thoughts about letting him participate in missions over enemy territory. Since he had some training in microbiology, he was assigned as a technician to Fleming's laboratory and set to work cleaning up what he found there. Apparently, dirty dishes and apparatus had been stacked up all over, and things must have been that way for a long time. Retelling his experiences after returning from the war, the student ventured the opinion that the *Penicillium* mold would not have grown in the laboratory and spread to the cocci culture if all the dishes had been washed regularly. Thus, penicillin might not have been discovered.

Not until 1937 was the real, useful antibiotic penicillin elaborated by a team of chemists and biologists at Oxford University (H. W. Florey, E. B. Chain, E. P. Abraham, N. G. Heatley). The first clinical use of penicillin was made 12 February 1941 on an Oxford policeman with a septic infection. For several years so little penicillin was available that any unchanged antibiotic had to be recovered from the urine of the patients and repurified for the next injection.

The term *penicillin* covers many drugs. Early in its investigation, more than seven similar but chemically different penicillins were found among the fermentation products. Since the chemistry of these penicillins emerged only slowly, a great deal of confusion accompanied the study of "penicillin." Clinically, these products were not equivalent either, and finally one of them, benzylpenicillin, was chosen as the most useful of these natural penicillins. It has become "the" penicillin of medicine. The drawback that it has to be given parenterally later led to the synthesis of orally active analogs that have replaced the natural products of the mold.

Fleming's original *Penicillium notatum* did not give a good yield of fermentation products. In 1944, R. D. Coghill at the Northern Regional Research Laboratories of the U.S. Department of Agriculture in Peoria, Illinois, isolated a strain of *Penicillium chrysogenum* from a moldy grapefruit and got a much higher yield of antibiotic from its fermentation. This strain has become the granddaddy of all the penicillin-producing molds all over the world. Another improvement was the introduction of cornsteep liquor as a nutrient for the fermenting mold. This is made by steeping cleaned corn grain in warm water containing 0.2 percent of sulfur dioxide, drawing off the water and concentrating under vacuum. It serves as a source of glucose and furnishes 1,000 times more penicillin than the older yeast extracts. Also, it became possible to "feed" the mold various chemicals that not only improved yields but led to the isolation of chemically modified penicillins—especially phenoxymethylpenicillin (penicillin V), which has some oral activity.

The difference between the penicillins is in the nature of the small chemical group ("side chain") always attached to the same main portion of the penicillin molecule, which is called 6-aminopenicillanic acid (6-APA). This substance became available on an industrial scale in 1959 and opened the floodgates to molecular modification of the penicillins. Any desired analog of penicillin could now be made in one simple chemical operation. The pharmaceutical industry lost no time making use of this opportunity. An estimated 10,000 penicillin analogs have been prepared and tested. From this research effort have come the modern penicillins. Some of them are orally active and need not be injected. Others overcame the resistance of bacteria that had sprung up to the earlier penicillins.

Some of them are active against a number of gram-negative pathogens, others against malarial plasmodia and other infectious organisms. Molecular modification has given the chemotherapist a selection of drugs for various infectious diseases.

All the penicillins have two things in common. First, they are relatively unstable chemicals, some more so than others. That is the reason the natural penicillins, the least stable ones, had to be injected rather than taken by mouth, because they broke down in the acidic stomach. This disadvantage has been remedied by careful chemical design of the side chains.

The second feature of all penicillins (and cephalosporins and other beta-lactam antibiotics) is their highly selective effect on the bacterial cell wall. Bacterial cells are enclosed in thin cell walls consisting of polysaccharides and proteins in tightly packed, cross-linked structures. The penicillins block the biosynthesis of these cell walls at one little point, the penultimate step of constructing the membrane network. Animal cells have no analogous membranes and are therefore immune to this interference by *beta*-lactam antibiotics.

THE CEPHALOSPORINS

After the publication of the penicillin studies, every pharmaceutical scientist, executive, and salesman was given a spatula and a box full of vials and was asked to dig up soil samples wherever they went. Samples were collected in New Jersey backyards, in summer gardens in New England, in forests in National Parks, in Venezuela, Western Australia, on Alpine slopes—all over. The samples were taken back to the lab, leached out, and worked up for potential antibiotic content. The yield from this aimless gamble was negligibly small, as was to the expected. Moreover, the same old antibiotics were isolated time and again from soils collected thousands of kilometers apart. Still, this exploratory search provided an opportunity for scientists and executives to travel to far-off places, to see the world using first-class airline tickets, and once in a while to return with a worthwhile soil sample. Professor Brotzu of the University of Cagliari on the Italian island of Sardinia collected sewage and grew an antibiotic-producing mold of the *Cephalosporium* species from this unappetizing source. He hit pay dirt: one of the components of the antibiotic broth was less active than benzylpenicillin but two to six times more active against gram-negative organisms. The Oxford group of microbiologists worked up the crude material and discovered that the new antibiotic had some similarities to penicillin, especially the beta-lactam structure, but it was more stable to acids. Molecular modification took over, and total syntheses of the complicated compounds were achieved, especially by the Nobelist Robert Woodward in 1966.

The cephalosporins from this work, which covered more than fifteen years, are useful in many previously untreatable infections. A breakthrough occurred when orally active cephalosporins and later long-acting cephalosporins were encountered. All of these are semisynthetic products.

An additional medical bonus was realized when the cephalosporins turned out to be much less allergenic than most penicillins. A total of circa 19 percent of all individuals do not tolerate penicillin. In the early days of antibiotics, penicillin used to be administered indiscriminately in large doses, since it was believed to be nontoxic. It is indeed nontoxic, but its potential for causing severe allergic reactions has led to greater caution in its use.

OTHER ANTIBIOTICS

Approximately seventy five antibiotics are in commercial production for clinical use. Many of them are semisynthetic. They are made from compounds derived from natural antibiotics and often represent clinical improvements over the natural product. Others are so similar in chemical structure and biological activity that they must be labeled as competitive drugs. As mentioned before, however, there is justification in having them available because some patients tolerate them better and some infectious bacteria are less liable to develop resistance to them.

Here, only a few important antibiotics of different chemical structure and a significant biological activity spectrum will be mentioned.

Not all antibiotics are used principally in clinical or veterinary medicine. It has been found that the growth and development of livestock is stunted by bacteria, especially in their alimentary canal. Antibiotics that kill such bacteria improve the development of domestic farm animals and are therefore incorporated routinely into the animal feed. However, in every bacterial population there is a small percentage of organisms resistant to this or that antibiotic. The antibiotic in the feed kills the bacteria that are affected by this chemical but leaves the resistant ones to multiply. If such resistant microorganisms get into the food chain, they can infect the human consumer of meat and then cannot be treated easily with existing antibiotics. Nevertheless, the livestock industry is loath to give up the advantages of antibiotic-enriched feed and uses one-half of all the antibiotics produced for its purposes. The greatest danger lies in resistance to the so-called broad-spectrum antibiotics, which are the favorite tools of the clinical chemotherapist because they free him from the task of determining what infectious agent he is dealing with.

One of the earliest and most unusual antibiotics was chloramphenicol, originally obtained from the fermentation of *Streptomyces venezuelae*. Its chemistry was described by Q. R. Bartz and his colleagues in 1948, and this was soon followed by a total synthesis by Mildred C. Rebstock. The synthesis was relatively simple, and now all the chloramphenicol is manufactured synthetically and no longer by fermentation.

Chloramphenicol is a broad-spectrum antibiotic with activity against gram-positive and gram-negative bacteria and rickettsiae. It also acts on large viruses, but its greatest value is as a curative drug in typhus and typhoid fever. One of its many side effects is bone marrow depression, which can lead to such blood disorders as aplastic anemia. Careful hematological control of patients can sidestep this danger.

In contrast to the penicillins and cephalosporins, which prevent the biosynthesis of bacterial cell walls, chloramphenicol inhibits bacterial protein synthesis from the amino acids. This kills bacteria but may also be the cause of the side effects of chloramphenicol on the cells of their mammalian hosts.

MACROLIDE ANTIBIOTICS

The macrolide antibiotics are produced by fermenting streptomycete strains that have been found in soil samples collected in all parts of the world. Those used in chemotherapy and in agriculture are erythromycin, leucomycin, oleandomycin, tylosin, and spiramycin. Chemically they are distinguished by large rings of carbon and oxygen atoms (lactone rings) attached to unusual sugars (deoxy sugars). Their biological activity extends mainly against gram-positive bacteria and *Mycoplasma*; they inhibit the biosynthesis of bacterial proteins at the stage of assembling amino acids to form the long peptide chains.

These antibiotics are being manufactured by competing pharmaceutical firms, whose drug insert pamphlets emphasize apparent advantages of the respective compounds. Physicians are influenced by these write-ups, and often prefer the first antibiotic of a group over the latecomers. Erythromycin and oleandomycin have similar antibacterial activity spectra, and a choice between them and others that act more or less on the same infections will be one of personal preference. Another factor will be drug allergies of patients, who sometimes tolerate one of a group of related drugs better than another.

Tylosin is promoted especially for the control of gram-positive bacteria and *Mycoplasma* infections of farm animals, such as respiratory diseases in poultry, dogs, and cats, and swine enteritis.

AMINOGLYCOSIDE ANTIBIOTICS

This group contains nitrogen-containing (aminocarbohydrate) sugar structures, several of them linked together. They inhibit gram-positive and gram-negative bacteria, including some hard to treat infections *(Pseudomonas aeruginosa)* and tubercle bacilli. Among these antibiotics are some of the earliest ones, streptomycin from *Streptomyces griseus* and dihydrostreptomycin. Streptomycin was the first effective agent for tuberculosis; but its toxicity for the eighth cranial nerve causes deafness, and its use has been abandoned in the U.S.A. The neomycins act similarly and are generally restricted to topical infections where they are not absorbed. Paramomycin, from *S. rimosus*, is also effective in amebic dysentery, shigellosis, and salmonellosis. The gentamycins, from *Micromonospora*, are good for *Pseudomonas* and *Proteus vulgaris* infections. The kanamycins, isolated from *S. kanamyceticus* in Japan, are especially suitable to combat urinary infections that resist other antibacterial agents.

TETRACYCLINES

Chlorotetracycline was obtained from *Streptomyces aureofaciens* by Duggart in 1947, and 5-hydroxytetracycline from *S. rimosus* by Finlay. Soon thereafter, tetracycline itself, the parent antibiotic of the others, was prepared by fermentation. These antibiotics are chemical derivatives of a four-ring system of carbon atoms called hydronaphthacene. Their biological activity is broad; they kill gram-positive bacteria, gram-negative cocci (but not gram-negative bacilli), spirochetes (that cause syphilis), tick-transmitted rickettsiae (Rocky Mountain spotted fever), and some larger viruses, including some involved in viral pneumonias. They are the most widely prescribed antibiotics next to the penicillins and the cephalosporins.

Chemical transformations of tetracycline have yielded many different derivatives, of which doxycycline should be mentioned. These semisynthetic antibiotics have provided competing manufacturers access to the lucrative tetracycline market, and some of them are indeed a little more effective and/or a little less toxic than others.

GRISEOFULVIN

Griseofulvin is obtainable from the metabolic fermentation of *Penicillium griseofulvum* and the mycelia of other *Penicillia*. It is orally active and is used for the systemic treatment of fungus infections.

LINCOMYCIN, NOVOBIOCIN

Lincomycin, from *Streptomyces lincolnensis*, has a unique chemical structure that was elucidated by a team of investigators at the Upjohn Company. It is highly effective against *Staphylococcus aureus* and other gram-positive bacteria that are spread in hospitals. It shows activity against these infections in patients who are allergic to penicillin.

Novobiocin, from several *Streptomyces* species, had been isolated numerous times from these fermentations and given different names. Its chemical structure is complex and consists of three separate sections joined together. Novobiocin is mainly active against staphylococcal and *Proteus*-infected skin lesions, urinary-tract infections, tonsillitis, and osteomyelitis.

THE RIFAMYCINS

The rifamycins are fermentation products of *Streptomyces mediterranei*. They inhibit gram-positive bacteria and mycobacteria. Their chemistry displays an elaborate large ring of carbon, nitrogen, and oxygen atoms that has taxed the ingenuity of some of the best organic chemists; the main contribution to this complicated problem was that of Piero Sensi in Milan, Italy. He also carried out extensive molecular modifications of the natural rifamycin antibiotics and arrived at a "long-shot" derivative, rifampicin. This compound has become an important antituberculous chemotherapeutic agent.

PEPTIDE ANTIBIOTICS

Over two hundred peptide antibiotics have been discovered, and the chemistry of some of the smaller peptides has been cleared up. As mentioned before in connection with peptide hormones, peptides are compounds composed of amino acids. The larger peptides with molecular weights over 6,000–10,000 are the proteins. The sequence of the amino acids in peptides determines their biological function. The shapes of the peptide molecules also affect the biological activity—whether the peptide will be a hormone or an antibiotic or just a biologically nondescript chemical. Some of the peptide antibiotics contain additional fragments: for example, the actinomycins, which are active against tumors. Other peptide antibiotics display circles of amino acids; they have cyclic structures. Examples are the bacitracins, valinomycin, the polymyxins, and gramicidin-S. Valinomycin can put a metal ion (potassium) in the center of its peptide ring and transport it across barriers, perhaps "stealing" potassium from some cells in this manner.

Most peptides cannot cross barriers of membranes easily, and therefore their antibiotic action is most useful in dermatology, where lotions or ointments are applied topically to burns, superficial ulcers, and other lesions.

14

Antiparasitic Drugs

MALARIA

Malaria is caused by protozoa of the genus *Plasmodium*, which have a life cycle partly in humans and partly in the female *Anopheles* mosquito. Four plasmodial species cause human malaria: *Plasmodium falciparum*, *P. vivax*, *P. malariae*, and *P. ovalis*. Similar parasites infect other mammals (*P. knowlesi* in monkeys), and *P. gallinaceum* occurs in fowl and reptiles. Falciparum malaria is also called malignant tertian malaria and, if untreated, is a life-threatening disease. Benign tertian malaria (every forty-eight hours) is caused by *P. vivax*; it leads to relapses for years after the primary infection. Quartan malaria (every seventy-two hours) is due to *P. malariae*; it is less severe than *vivax* Malaria but can persist for many years.

Malaria is characterized by attacks of very high fever that leave the patient prostrate and debilitated. The disease is endemic in hot humid climates conducive to the development of the insect vector, the *Anopheles* mosquito. That does not mean that people in more moderate climates need not be concerned about malaria. It has been stated that the Roman civilization declined because the population was weakened by malaria. In Charleston, South Carolina, and New Orleans, malaria was prevalent until recent times. The decisive control of malaria is achieved by a systematic campaign against the mosquito vector with insecticides. The introduction of DDT (chlorophenothane) by Paul Müller in the late 1930s did more for the eradication of malaria in Southern Europe and North America than any other measure. In Southern Asia, South America, and tropical Africa the topography and economics of the region have not made these attempts at mosquito control effective, and worldwide hundreds of millions of cases of malaria are still counted.

The plasmodia undergo sexual development in the gut of the female *Anopheles* mosquito and accumulate in its salivary gland. When the mosquito takes a blood meal, it injects a plasmodial spore (sporozoite) into its victim. The sporozoites rapidly assemble in the liver, where they begin an asexual division. No symptoms of the disease appear for eight to twelve days. Plasmodial cell division is complex; only some of its stages will be listed. The plasmodial cells first divide outside of blood corpuscles; the liver cells in which they develop rupture and empty a form called merozoites into the bloodstream. The merozoites infect red blood corpuscles and invade them. The blood cells rupture, empty merozoites, and these reinvade new erythrocytes. This causes a relapse. A few merozoites now decide to multiply by a sexual process and for this purpose become male and female gametocytes. When the host is bitten again by a mosquito, these male and female cells enter the stomach of the insect, get fertilized, and produce egg-type cells, which go to the salivary glands, rupture, and release the sporozoites that infect the next victim of the mosquito.

The simplest way to stop the life cycle of the plasmodia would be to kill the sporozoites that enter the human body with the bite of an infected mosquito. This has not yet been possible. An anti-sporozoite vaccine might be the best measure to cope with the start of the infection. Very recently, antibodies to sporozoite proteins have been made, and the hope has been expressed that a vaccine is on the way. Until the formidable difficulties of this undertaking are overcome, one has to interrupt the plasmodial life cycle at other stages.

A malarial patient has no other choice but chemotherapy. The time-honored drug from the seventeenth century to the recent past has been quinine. Quinine is the principal alkaloid of the cinchona tree. Its chemistry is complicated, and attempts have been made repeatedly to peel out the molecular features that endow the alkaloid with suppressive activity. This has been the guiding thought in much of the antimalarial research. This work experienced three climactic peaks. The first one came during World War I when the German pharmaceutical industry tried to synthesize drugs that might replace quinine, because quinine was no longer accessible from its Dutch East Indies cinchona plantations. This effort was only partially successful but pointed the way for future researches. The second phase of antimalarial research occurred during the next military adventure of the human race in World War II, after the Japanese invasion of Southeast Asia and the renewed loss of the sources of quinine. From that massive and much more sophisticated research in the United States, the U.S.S.R., and Britain arose almost all the antimalarial drugs that are in use today.

The third wave of antimalarial research arrived under the sponsorship of the U.S. Army during its ill-fated adventure in Vietnam. Here plasmodia resistant to the available drugs were encountered, and new chemicals had to be invented to overcome this resistance. In spite of many successes, the problem of chemotherapy of malaria has not yet been solved completely.

Antimalarial drugs are tested in infected animals. For decades, avian plasmodial infections in chickens and turkey chicks were used, but after World War II, an organism *(Plasmodium berghei)* was discovered that could be used in mice. Since then, in the hands of Leon Rane of the University of Miami, antimalarial tests have become faster and more efficient. Follow-up studies are made in Rhesus monkeys infected with *P. knowlesi* and in volunteers bitten by infected *Anopheles* mosquitoes.

The researches in the United States and in continental Europe took their lead from one of the structural sections of the quinine molecule, a ring system called quinoline. To this was attached a nitrogen-carbon-nitrogen chain of atoms, and the resulting compounds showed potent antimalarial activity both in bird malarias and in clinical malarias. Only the drugs that survived the selection from 30,000 candidate compounds will be mentioned. Chloroquine has remained one of the most effective suppressive antimalarials. It can be taken orally to ward off the symptoms of infections by the schizont forms of the plasmodia. Primaquine is an effective drug against the sexual forms of the parasite. Quinacrine (Atebrin) was used widely by the military to keep troops free of relapses; it has the disadvantage of dyeing the skin yellow. During the U.S. Army's research effort in the Vietnamese conflict, a quinine analog called mefloquine was developed by R. E. Lutz at the University of Virginia. It is singularly active against falciparum plasmodia that have become resistant to chloroquine.

The quinoline antimalarials become layered between helical turns of nucleic acid and prevent the uncoiling needed for initiation of cell division of plasmodial parasites.

In Britain the enzyme dihydrofolate reductase was found to be needed by the plasmodia for building their nucleic acids in their cells, and therefore pyrimidine analogs were constructed that might have a chance to counteract this enzyme, since pyrimidines are among the products made under its influence. The two drugs, selected from huge numbers of analogs, were chlorguanide and especially pyrimethamine (Daraprim). Investigators in China isolated in 1972 an unorthodox drug from a traditional Chinese medicinal herb, *Artemisia annua* L., which had been known for almost 2,000 years as Quinghao. The drug, quinghaosu (or artemisin), is apparently an effective antimalarial.

DRUGS FOR AMEBIASIS

Amebiasis is caused by the infection with a parasitic, microscopic, one-celled protozoan called *Entamoeba histolytica*. This parasite has five stages in its life cycle, all of which occur in the human intestine. The infection is transferred by amebal cysts, either in contaminated food or water, in cyst-containing clothing, or directly from an infected person. The cyst passes into the small intestine, it ruptures, and the contents disperse as a stage called metacysts. Each of these metacysts form trophozoite organisms that grow in size, invade tissues, and form lesions by digesting the tissues of the host.

Further down in the intestine the trophozoites mature to cysts through intermediary stages and are now ready to infect the next victim.

Amebiasis is characterized by dysentery and liver abscesses. It used to be regarded as a tropical disease but has also been found in more moderate climates. It is fourteenth among diseases as a cause of illness and thirteenth as a cause of death worldwide. Although the incidence of amebiasis is highest in the tropics, at least 5 percent of the U.S. population is infected. The most apparent cause of the spread of amebiasis is poor sanitation, lack of pure drinking water, and lack of sewage facilities, rather than geographic latitude.

Various laboratory animals can be infected with amebae and drugs can be tested against these infections. Both in animal models and in the clinical trials of antiamebic agents, the major difficulties are in dealing with intestinal versus liver infections.

The oldest amebicidal compounds are the ipecac alkaloids. The principal alkaloid is emetine. As its name indicates, it causes vomiting, a property for which powdered ipecac root has been used for centuries. This toxic action is minimized by concurrent administration of a sedative, and then emetine can unfold its antiamebic action. Since emetine shows a number of other bothering side effects, molecular modification by medicinal chemists has tried to point up the antiamebic action. Only one of the hundreds of variations tried has some clinical advantages over emetine; this drug is called 2-dehydroemetine.

Other natural plant products used successfully as amebicides in humans are glaucarubin from the bark of *Simarouba glauca* and several antibiotics, especially paramomycin (from a *Streptomyces* strain). Paramomycin inhibits the incorporation of amino acids into bacterial proteins.

Purely synthetic compounds have been screened as antiamebic agents in vast numbers, and a few have been introduced as clinical drugs for amebiasis. Among them are clamoxyquin pamoate, which is not only an effective amebicide but also subdues *Shigella* infections and giardiasis, an infection caused by *Giardia lamblia* that is acquired from drinking water in eastern Europe. More or less equivalent is iodochlorhydroxyquin. This drug has been advertised as a prophylactic agent against travelers' diarrhea under the name of Entero-Vioform, but its effectiveness for such purposes is in question. The antimalarial drug amodiaquine has shown good prophylactic activity against amebiasis. It has been overshadowed by a similar chemical agent, bialamicol, which is specific for amebiasis and its complications.

A unique and very reliable antiamebic drug is metronidazole. It was created as an antitrichomonal agent, and its amebicidal potency was discovered during additional screening against other protozoa.

Arsenical drugs, investigated by Paul Ehrlich before 1910, have lost territory to less toxic agents, but one of them, carbarsone, is still used in the chemotherapy of amebiasis.

Little has been said about the mechanism of action of clinically useful amebicides. The reason is that not much is known. Most of them interfere with various stages of protein synthesis in the ameba.

OTHER PROTOZOAN DISEASES

Protozoa other than malarial plasmodia and *Entamoeba histolytica* are also causes of major diseases of man and domestic animals. The two most serious of these diseases are trypanosomiasis and leishmaniasis.

Trypanosomiasis is an infection spread over tropical zones of our earth. In Africa, *Trypanosoma gambiense* and *T. rhodesiense* cause sleeping sickness in man. These microorganisms are elongated, rapidly moving cells. They spend part of their life cycle in the tsetse fly *(Glossina)*, which transmits them to man and other mammals through its bite. Damage caused to livestock by trypanosomiasis has denied large land areas in Africa to all domestic animals except poultry. Antelopes and other wild game serve as reservoirs of trypanosomes. Again, as in the case of mosquito control for malaria and yellow fever, broad-spectrum contact insecticides offer the best prevention of trypanosomiasis. In South and Central America, *Trypanosoma cruzi*, transmitted by another tsetse fly, causes Chagas' disease in humans, mostly in children. In animals the disease is called nagana; it is caused by *T. brucei*. Other forms of animal trypanosomiasis in South America are mal de caderas, transmitted by bloodsucking flies, and sura, transmitted by vampire bats. All the trypanosomes can be maintained in artificial infections in laboratory rodents and are thereby amenable to chemotherapeutic evaluation.

Early chemotherapeutic studies of trypanosomiasis relied on various azo dyes in Ehrlich's laboratory. Because these dyes colored the host tissues, noncoloring analogs were soon sought. In carefully executed studies of molecular modification, those sections of the dyestuff molecules that convey dyestuff character (chromophore groups) were exchanged for noncoloring portions. The outcome was suramin, which is still a valuable drug for African sleeping sickness.

Another product of that pre-1920 period was an arsenical drug, tryparsamide, still in use against Gambian sleeping sickness despite its considerable toxicity. An arsenical, melarsoprol, developed later, is more valuable as a chemotherapeutic trypanocide. Stilbamidine and homidium are two chemically different drugs used in veterinary medicine. No permanent success has been scored in the treatment of South American Chagas' disease.

The parasites causing leishmaniasis are *Leishmaniae*. These organisms are stored in dogs and gerbils and are transferred to humans by the bite of sand flies. At one time the insect vectors and the disease were found in the coastal regions of South Carolina. Clinical manifestations of leishmaniasis are oriental sore, espundia, and Kalaazar. The parasites can be established in hamsters for chemotherapeutic studies.

The chemotherapy of leishmaniasis leaves much to be desired. A number of compounds containing the heavy-metal element antimony are the traditional drugs for this infection but antimonials, arsenicals, and other heavy-metal compounds are beset with toxicity. If nothing better turns up in a search for antiparasitic drugs, agents with established activity against other protozoa and parasites are screened. In this way, an antimalarial, cycloguanil, was found to have activity against South American leishmaniases.

The most aggravating protozoan disease of women in the temperature zones is trichomoniasis, a venereal disease caused by direct sexual contact. Its causative microbial organism is *Trichomonas vaginalis*. A similar parasite, *T. foetus*, invades the genital tract of cows and leads to sterility and abortion in these farm animals.

The leading drug for trichomoniasis is metronidazole, the end product of long searches in the U.S. and in France. After the discovery of the antitrichomonal activity of metronidazole, the drug was screened against every protozoan and other parasite. Among the conditions in which it is of value is giardiasis, a protozoan infection caused by drinking water contaminated with *Giardia intestinalis*. Metronidazole is also amebicidal.

There are numerous additional protozoan infections but since they primarily affect domestic animals, they will not be treated here. Their chemotherapy is a problem for successful agriculture and production of healthy animals for human consumption.

ANTHELMINTICS

One third of the human race harbors parasitic worms. One usually thinks of worm infections as tropical diseases, but over 40 million Americans are also victims of parasitic worms. These worms are also a threat to all domestic and farm animals and cause serious problems to animal breeders. The most widespread human worm infestations (helminthiases) are schistosomiasis, ascariasis, and hookworm diseases. The most troublesome helminthiases of animals are fluke and roundworm infections.

Most people are aware of tapeworms (cestodes), which inhabit the intestinal tract of the host and rob the host of nutrients. They are ingested with infected diets. Fish tapeworm *(Diphyllobothrium latum)* develops in animals and people that consume raw fish. Beef tapeworm *(Taenia saginata)* and pork tapeworm *(T. solium)* are acquired from meat in the form of worm larvae. Other tapeworms of humans are the dwarf tapeworm *(Hymenolepis nana)* and *Echinococcus granulosis*.

Flukes (trematodes) are primitive worms. The larvae of the lung fluke *(Paragonimus westermani)* enter the body in a diet of infested crabs. The liver fluke *(Clonorchis sinensis)* and other similar flukes are acquired from infected fish, and the intestinal fluke *(Fasciolopsis buski)* from edible water plants that harbor encysted larvae of this animal.

Three species of schistosomes exist as male and female worms that invade the blood vessels of the peritoneum and other mesenteric membranes, with symptoms arising in the intestines, liver, and spleen. Other forms of schistosomiasis are caused by *Schistosoma haematobium*, which lodges in the bladder, the anus, the kidneys, and the female genitals. Man acquires schistosomes directly from free-living cercarial forms of the worms in water. The cercariae invade the skin and hence many internal organs, where they undergo a sexual life cycle. The eggs of the female worms are excreted with stool and urine, hatch in water to organisms that invade snails, and there change again to cercariae, ready to infect other human hosts. Many attempts have been made to kill the snail vectors with molluscocides, both inorganic and organic chemicals; however, the extensive irrigation canals and the habit of standing in water while planting rice in many tropical and semitropical countries has not been able to make snail control a success. Therefore, chemotherapy of established infections is of great importance. *Schistosoma mansoni* can be grown in mice and *S. japonicum* in monkeys for the evaluation of antischistosomal drugs.

Nematodes (roundworms) look more like real "worms." They include hookworms, the whipworm, and the pinworm. They invade the human skin or are acquired in the diet; *Trichinella spiralis*, which causes trichinosis, is ingested with poorly cooked, infected pork.

It is obvious that such a variety of parasitic worms will require a variety of chemotherapeutic drugs to combat the often terrible diseases caused by the worms. Some small worms are so translucent that their internal organs can be studied from the outside. Others are covered with tough membranes, and their organs are differentiated extensively. The fact that the vectors of the worms are associated with careless and unsanitary life habits and with poverty contributes to the difficulty of chemotherapeutic intervention. In addition, no persuasion or education can be applied to domestic and farm animals that get worm diseases in the normal course of their life. Cats, dogs, cattle, sheep, horses, etc., need frequent deworming or anthelmintic chemotherapy for economic as well as sanitary reasons. A large effort has therefore gone into the study of anthelmintic drugs. The enormous evolutionary difference between the parasitic worm and the higher-animal host would point to the possibility of a comfortable margin of toxicity of drugs for the two types of organisms. However, worms, animals, and humans depend on the same fundamental sources of energy and on the same or at least very similar enzymes for the basic reactions of their processes. If a drug inhibits a controlling enzyme in a worm, it may be expected that it will also affect the analogous enzyme system in a host. Therefore, drugs for helminthiases share the potential toxicity with many drugs for other types of parasitic invasions.

This is demonstrated in drugs for tapeworm diseases. These are caused by several species of *Hymenolepis* and *Taenia*. One of the oldest drugs, still in use in spite of its toxicity, is extract of male fern *(Aspidium oleoresin)*, which contains such taenicidal compounds as filixic acid. Several other tapeworm-removing medicines have been discovered by screening in small (mice) and larger animals (cats, dogs). Among them are the old antimalarial quinacrine, the phenolic derivative dichlorophen, the salicylic acid derivative niclosamide, and the antibiotic paromomycin.

In the trematode worm infection schistosomiasis, one has to combat various human blood flukes of the genus *Schistosoma*. Originally treated with the objectionable antimonial agent tartar emetic, schistosomiasis is still treated with antimony compounds such as stibophen and stibocaptate, but these injectable drugs have been replaced by orally active, metal-free schistosomicides that are less toxic. Two of these are lucanthone and hycanthone; the latter is a mammalian metabolite of lucanthone, and administration of lucanthone is therefore, after delay for oxidative metabolism in the body, more or less equivalent to taking hycanthone directly. Another drug, niridazole, is effective against several but not all species of *Schistosoma*. This specificity also limits the effectiveness of the other antischistosomal agents, and careful morphological diagnosis of the parasite should determine the drug for prescription in chemotherapy. Since over 300,000 persons are afflicted by schistosomiasis worldwide, early diagnosis is a serious problem.

These numbers assume even more frightening proportions in the case of the estimated 200 million people suffering from filariasis and the 30 million who have gone blind from onchocerciasis. Other nematode infections are found in equally high percentages of the rural population in warm climates: 20 percent are suffering from ascariasis, 25 percent from ancylostomiasis, and 10 percent from oxyuriasis. In spite of major research efforts in a few institutions and industrial laboratories, chemotherapeutic work on nematode infections has not been one of the major competitive programs because the poverty-stricken patients cannot be expected to return the enormous research investments. It is different in the husbandry fields, where nematodes wreak damage. When properly treated, the cured animals compensate for the cost of the necessary research expenditures. Since this volume hopes to explain the origin and mode of action of drugs used in clinical medicine, emphasis will be given to such agents.

Filariasis occurs in Africa, China, India, Japan, the East and West Indies, and Central America. The most important nematodes causing the infections are *Wuchereria bancrofti*, *W. malayi*, and *Onchocerca volvulus*. These worms go through a life cycle of which one phase is called micro-filariae. These develop into infecting larvae in mosquitoes and are transmitted by the insect to the mammalian host. There they migrate into the lymph vessels and continue a cycle of sexual reproduction, resulting in adult worms. If repeated heavy infection occurs, the larvae and adult worms can block lymph vessels and give rise to such swellings as elephantiasis. The preferred chemotherapeutic agent for the removal of microfilariae is diethylcarbamazine, discovered by S. Kushner and his colleagues. The destruction of the microfilariae especially in loiasis (*Loa loa* infection) may cause allergic reactions. This can be controlled by giving smaller doses of the drug initially or by coadministering an antihistaminic agent. Diethylcarbamazine is not very effective against onchocerciasis (*O. volvulus* infections). This is controlled better by suramin.

Hookworm disease responds well to biphenium, which kills *Ancylostoma duodenale*. Most patients suffer from multiple intestinal-worm infections, often infestations by *Ascaris lumbricoides* and *Trichostrongylus orientalis*. In such cases thiabendazole is of value. Thiabendazole has become primarily an agent for the control of gastrointestinal nematode infections of ruminant animals.

Ascariasis and oxyuriasis are treated with a simple chemical called piperazine. It is highly active, virtually nontoxic, and cheap. It was discovered by screening after trials in unrelated rheumatic disorders. Oxyuriasis is caused by *Oxyuris* (pinworms); it is the most common worm disease of American school children. Piperazine is the most effective drug for this disease. Coadministration of another anthelmintic called pyrantel, developed in the Pfizer Research Laboratories, clears up concurrent ascaris infections. Thiabendazole is also of value.

The Belgian drug levamisole is a broad-spectrum anthelmintic active against a large number of pathogenic nematodes in thirteen hosts, including humans. It is not effective in intestinal *Trichuris* infections.

Anthelmintic drugs act by depriving the various life stages of the worms of essential enzyme systems. Manipulation of low dosages and coadministration of low (barely effective) doses of two or more drugs with overlapping activities offers the best hope for minimizing systemic toxicity, with its inherent unwanted side effects.

Many anthelmintics with some activity against exotic worm diseases have been omitted from this discussion because few physicians in the developed countries would encounter these infections and learn how to treat them. Those doctors who do will probably try out the existing newer anthelmintics or reach back to some older ones if they are still available, and they may have to undertake a careful differential diagnosis if their patients have acquired the worm infestation during a trip to unsanitary regions. Then it will be necessary to search the literature for records of clinically successful drugs for the disease at hand.

ANTIFUNGAL AGENTS

For the purposes of the chemotherapist, the term *fungi* covers both yeasts and molds that attach themselves to tissues and draw their nutrients from the cells of their host. The diseases are called mycoses. There are three types of mycotic diseases: (1) superficial contagious skin infections (dermatophytoses); (2) candidiasis, also called moniliasis, which causes lesions on the skin and mucous membranes, but can also invade internal organs; (3) deep mycoses that are not contagious but invade the skin, lungs, lymph, and other internal systems; they can be sand borne, or arise from contact with fungi on vegetation or other objects, or from diets contaminated with saprophytic molds or mushrooms.

A fourth class, not strictly fungus infections, comprises the actinomycoses. They infect the lung and other organs. They are caused by Actinomycetales, an order of organisms between molds and bacteria.

Fungal diseases had been known before the early bacteriologists (Pasteur, Koch) recognized bacteria as causes of many infections. They are assuming greater importance today, not only because more cases of serious primary mycoses are being diagnosed, but because systemic fungal infections so often lodge in patients with neoplastic diseases and lead to the death of the individual.

Superficial fungi use keratin as their substrate; however, the fundamental biochemical reactions—the oxidative transformations yielding energy for all cells, with the same overall enzymes as in other cells—are also used by fungal life processes. Consequently, drugs for fungistasis must be found by trial and error among chemicals that inhibit cellular life in general.

Salts of fatty acids have long been claimed to be fungistatic, but their value is not beyond dispute. The best is undecylenic acid, an 11-carbon unsaturated acid. It is effective in bringing to a halt the spread of *tinea pedis* (athlete's foot), but in other dermatomycoses on the head and in the hair it is of less value.

Other synthetic substances with a broader antifungal spectrum include miconazole, a rather nontoxic drug whose chemistry is similar to that of antihistaminic agents. Indeed, several antihistaminics have minor antifungal activities. A number of superficial fungal diseases that affect the skin and mucous membranes such as the vagina respond well to miconazole. Other topical fungal infections such as those caused by *Trichophyton* species are treatable with tolnaftate. Compounds that withdraw metal ions from essential fungal life processes can stop the reproduction of some fungi; iodochlorhydroxyquin is one of these products. It is still used in *Candida* and *Monilia* infections but is giving way to antifungal antibiotics.

Most of these antibiotics are prescription drugs because their indiscriminate application in insufficient amounts to inflamed membranes might lead to drug-resistant fungi. People suffering from minor fungal skin infections often want to relieve the itching and other discomfort without consulting an expensive physician. They turn to older, less effective over-the-counter salves and ointments, that may or may not work on their undiagnosed skin lesions. Among these are salicylic acid ointment, acrisorcin cream (it may produce hives and blisters), chlordantoin (for candidiasis), and several old dyestuffs that have survived a no-longer-deserved reputation of antifungal activity.

The modern dermatologist prefers to try antibiotics for the treatment of both superficial and deep-seated mycotic infections. Griseofulvin, a product of *Penicillium griseofulvum*, is active orally and diffuses to the site of skin and hair lesions. It has low toxicity. Griseofulvin is bound to the lipids of the fungal cells. It is effective in fungal diseases of the skin, hair, and nails caused by *Microsporum*, *Trichophyton*, and *Epidermophyton* species. Nystatin is an antibiotic from *Streptomyces noursei*; amphotericin B is another one from *S. nodosus*. These two belong chemically to the class of polyene antibiotics that features large rings of carbon atoms interrupted by some oxygen atoms. They bind to the sterol lipids of yeasts and fungi, disrupt their cell membranes, and allow small nutrient molecules to leak out. Nystatin is less toxic than amphotericin B; they are both effective against a wide variety of pathogenic fungi and yeasts. Nystatin is the preferred drug for *Candida* infections, while amphotericin B can overcome internal mycoses that were fatal prior to the introduction of this antibiotic.

15

Antiseptics and Disinfectants

The air we breathe and the water we bathe in are loaded with "germs," i.e., bacteria, fungi, and other microbes. The walls and floors of our buildings, the clothes we wear, and the dishes we serve our food on are equally covered with microorganisms. So are our bodies even if we wash them thoroughly. That is why surgeons scrub and have their hands protected before an operation. Some of these microorganisms are harmless, some are pathogenic or destructive because they feed on tissues and materials on which they alight. If we wish to live hygienically and protect our dwellings and surroundings from pathogens, we must cleanse ourselves and the objects around us with chemicals that inhibit or kill the damaging microbes. Even nonpathogenic bacteria and fungi must decompose perspiration and fibers in order to find nutrients; they produce offending odors and discolorations. A large industry has been built up to manufacture chemicals, soaps, and preparations to combat microbial processes on inanimate surfaces and on mammalian and human skins. The advertisements for such chemicals point out unhesitatingly the damaging consequences of *not* using those products. Commercial television and Sunday sections of newspapers depend on the advertisements for their economic survival.

Sterilization means destruction of all forms of life, whether it be that of vegetative cells of bacteria, of bacterial or other microbial spores, or of viruses. Long exposure of surgical instruments to sterilizing solutions at high temperatures may achieve sterilization, but larger objects cannot be fully cleansed of microbial cells. Such objects as floors, walls, toilets, etc., can only be disinfected. Disinfectants will kill most vegetative forms of microorganisms but not bacterial or fungal spores, and will not be expected to remove viruses from inanimate objects. Sanitizers must reduce bacteria to levels acceptable to public health rules. They are of significance in cleansing plates and cups in restaurants and in cleaning up machinery in food-processing plants. If chemicals only inhibit the multiplication ("growth") of microbes, they are microbistatic (bacteriostatic, virustatic, etc.). If they apparently kill the microbes, they are called microbicidal (bactericidal, virucidal, fungicidal, etc.). Such -cidal agents, when applied to living tissue, are termed antiseptics: for example, mouthwashes and deodorant soaps.

In the commercial disinfectants and antiseptics, the active ingredients are mixed with detergents, antifoam agents, dispersants, aerosols, and coloring matter. Occasionally more than one active ingredient is present. The antibacterial potency is determined by the killing power of the agent for a number of representative microorganisms and is compared to an arbitrarily chosen standard. For example, a certain concentration of phenol (carbolic acid) is given a value of 1.0, and the dilution of the disinfectant to be tested that kills test bacteria in a certain number of minutes is assigned a comparative value. The bacteria that must be killed under these conditions are *Salmonella typhosa* or *S. choleraesius*, *Staphylococcus aureus*, and *Proteus vulgaris*. The standard fungus is *Trichophyton interdigitale*. Other tests measure the comparative activity against some bacterial spores, tubercle bacilli, and specific viruses against which effectiveness is being claimed.

There are roughly the following types of disinfectants: phenolic compounds that are acidic and go into solution in alkali; quaternary ammonium compounds that are water-soluble ionic materials; oxidizing agents such as hydrogen peroxide; volatile alkylating agents such as ethylene oxide, formaldehyde, and propiolactone, which can sterilize inanimate objects by fumigation; chlorine, chloramines, and hypochlorites, used in swimming pools and in household sanitizers; and miscellaneous substances that can be used dermatologically and border on topical chemotherapeutic agents.

Phenol (carbolic acid), used by Lister in 1867, is only of historical interest because of its toxic, necrotizing properties. A number of related compounds, obtained from coal tar or by complete synthesis, have been more useful. They contain chlorine or various carbon chains (alkyl groups). Among those in use in antisepsis are chlorocresol, chloroxylenol, metacresyl acetate, hexylresorcinol, hexachlorophen, and several similar products. Some of these are used as skin disinfectants, in the outer ear, in mouthwashes, and in dermatology. Oxine is a phenol derived from a nitrogen-containing system called quinoline. It can bind metal ions and by removing them, deprives microbes of ions that are essential to their life processes.

If an atom of nitrogen is combined with four organic chemical radicals (R), and if one of these radicals is long enough to make the compound look like a soap, you get quaternary ammonium salts ("quats") that have potent antiseptic activity. They were first made by Hartmann and Kägi in 1928. They are not without drawbacks, the most serious being that some bacteria become resistant to them. Some quats are also effective antiviral disinfectants. Among them are cetylpyridinium chloride, benzethonium, and benzalkonium.

Chlorine and hypochlorites dissolve in water to give a certain amount of hypochlorous acid, which kills microbes by oxidation. Since other organic matter (plant debris, etc.) is also oxidized, it is necessary to clean the water before applying a source of hypochlorous acid. A number of organic chloramines such as halazone, chlorosuccinimide, and chlorinated isocyanuric acids are more versatile agents for the release of chlorine. They are effective wound disinfectants but may be toxic when ingested.

Chlorine is not the only bactericidal halogen. Iodine tincture acts similarly in solution, owing its activity to the combination of iodine with bacterial proteins.

A number of peroxides, perborates, permanganate salts, and other oxidizing agents are used as disinfectants on various body surfaces. They oxidize (burn up) components of bacterial membranes and other proteins.

The stiff competition for the disinfectant market has given rise to many other compounds with good, moderate, or inferior antimicrobial activity. The U.S. Food and Drug Administration and the Department of Agriculture keep a watchful eye on these products and try to protect the consumer from ineffective and toxic substances.

16

Peoples' Attitudes toward Drugs

There are people who pride themselves on "never" taking any drugs whatsoever. This is to be recommended during pregnancy, because some drugs can traverse the placenta and may cause adverse or even dangerous effects in the fetus. In all other conceivable conditions, however, not taking a drug when it might alleviate a disease or discomfort is unjustifiable. Religious fanatics may deny themselves the comfort of medications, but normal, rational individuals should never consider falling into that trap.

The other extreme encompasses people who take too many drugs. Some even take every drug in sight, and others take a drug because it was given to them free or sold as a bargain. This holds not only for vitamins, although they are first in line. One elderly woman we knew lined up twenty-four capsules and tablets on the breakfast table and washed these pretty, multicolored chemicals down with another drug product, coffee. She had collected her medications quite simply. Her physician prescribed three or four for her, but when she bought them she was assailed by doubts. Would they really work? Would it not be better to ask for a second opinion about her condition? Insurance would pay most of her bill, and so she saw a second—and finally a third—physician. These doctors diagnosed the same illness as the first one but prescribed different brands of the same medication. They also recommended a few vitamin capsules, and that is how she ended up with all those pills. The outcome was that she ingested three times the therapeutic dose of each medication. No wonder she landed in a hospital with toxicity symptoms from these overdoses.

This case is not unusual. The high cost of visits to a physician drives thousands of patients everywhere to attempt self-medication with over-the-counter, nonprescription drugs. Catastrophic intoxication is avoided only because those over-the-counter drugs are often not very effective anyway. This does not protect sensitive individuals from allergic reactions to the drug. It does not eliminate the danger of overmedication in attempts to commit suicide.

All this illustrates the fact that many patients do not comply with their physician's prescriptions and directions. Some patients just will not take the prescribed drugs at all, for whatever reason—unwillingness to obey orders; adherence to Christian Science, which shuns drugs; or because their bridge partner or beauty parlor operator has warned them of side effects of the drug. Others want to save the expense of buying the prescription—and some drugs are indeed very expensive.

Physicians are aware of drug interactions but in years past did not adequately focus on such dangers. The best advice on drug interactions can be obtained from a knowledgeable pharmacist, some of whom now hold a Doctor of Pharmacy degree. A pharmacist who can supply such information can be as important to the patient as a physician.

Drugs may interact with each other by influencing each other's metabolism, absorption, etc. For example, phenobarbital can stimulate the oxidative destruction of several unrelated drugs and thereby make them less long-lasting and less effective. Anticoagulants are made less effective by barbiturates and a spate of other, unrelated drugs. When such drugs are used concurrently, blood clotting may occur. It is therefore imperative to follow a physician's careful directions in such cases.

Obviously, two drugs that have the same type of activity should not be taken simultaneously unless toxicity from large doses of either of these drugs is to be minimized. Many patients heap one "painkiller" on top of another, which may induce depression and other unwanted side effects. Two drugs that have opposite activity should not be administered together either. Thus, vitamin K, which promotes blood coagulation, will nullify the action of an anticoagulant.

Not all harmful interactions arise from two drugs that interfere with each other; dietary factors also play a role. The most famous case is that of cheddar cheese, red wine, or bananas and the antidepressant monoamine oxidase inhibitors. Those foods contain a biogenic amine called tyramine, which raises the blood pressure. Ordinarily, tyramine is destroyed rapidly by the enzyme monoamine oxidase, but if this enzyme is held in check by the monoamine oxidase inhibitors, tyramine may lead to a dangerous rise in blood pressure. Likewise, while taking an antibiotic, it would be foolish to include vitamins and other nutrients in one's diet that promote the essential life processes of the pathogens. Tetracycline loses its antibacterial activity when taken with milk or other calcium-containing foods because it forms an insoluble product with calcium.

On the other hand, combination of several drugs in one tablet may not only be convenient but also pharmacologically justified. Many anticancer drugs must be taken in doses verging on overt toxicity if they are to be effective. By mixing lower doses of three anticancer drugs and attacking tumor growth by three different biological routes, some of the toxic side effects of the individual components of the mixture can be minimized.

Some drugs, when taken in excessive doses or over long periods of time, can induce symptoms of chronic toxicity that may well be called drug-induced diseases. A considerable percentage of patients seeking admission to hospitals are victims of such drug diseases. Reversing the chronic effects of a drug is difficult if not impossible. Since all drugs are tested for chronic toxicity in laboratory animals before being admitted to clinical usage, experienced physicians will be able to adjust prescriptions in a manner that promises to avoid such incidents.

The physician is regarded by patients as a dual person. He must be competent in diagnosing and treating the disease and in prescribing the most up-to-date and effective and the least toxic drugs. Most patients require a second quality in their doctor, whether he be a primary family practitioner or a specialist. They want him or her to be a sympathetic, comforting parent figure, emanating professional authority *and* compassion. This is demanding a good deal from a physician who sees and treats twenty and sometimes fifty or more patients every day. However, it is the physician's duty to explain the diagnosis to the patient, prescribe adequate medication, and advise about side effects or even failures of the drug prescribed. The physician should also make it clear when and how long a drug should be taken. Elderly patients, especially those with little education, may stop taking an antibiotic as soon as they are free from fever, and will invite a relapse if they interrupt the treatment before all pathogens have been killed. A factual attitude toward all drugs without prejudice will do much to help in the drug therapy of a disease. This factual attitude should include the hope that a given drug will do the task expected of it, but that the drugs, like all the creations of human brains, cannot be expected to be perfect.

QUACKERY

The horse-drawn medicine cart, gaily painted and decorated, has been a cherished American tradition in the same league as the circus coming to town. The driver of the cart was a combination comedian, huckster, self-appointed health adviser, and fake. Crowds greeted his visit and men and women alike succumbed to his hard-sell advertising of snake-bite oil, hair tonics for balding heads, rejuvenating nostrums, aphrodisiacs, deworming medicines, and backache liniments.

The blandishments of these unauthorized "doctors" and the ineffectiveness of their medications were the direct cause of the Pure Food and Drug Act that the U.S. Congress passed in 1906. This legislation abolished most, although not all, outright quackery that had been foisted on the public by medical swindlers in a shameless manner for centuries.

Control of any new legislation takes time, and even today, eighty years after it was enacted, the public is still confronted by a few unscrupulous manipulators who attempt to extort money from sick and despairing patients and their families. The advertisements of pain relievers in the news media are now couched in careful sentences designed to stay on the razor edge of legally allowed language, but the average listener, suffering from pain, barely ever sees through the line dividing truth from deceit. The same holds for the ointments that are said to relieve the pain and itching caused by hemorrhoids, the adhesive that holds dentures firmly in place, and all the other concoctions that pay for the broadcasting time of the evening news.

Such extravagances are of minor importance, and reasonable people will smile at them and chalk them up to the perverse desire to believe in something that can barely be true. The Romans had a proverb for that: *Mundus vult decipi, ergo decipiatur* ("The world wants to be deceived, therefore let it be deceived"). Only when health or recovery from a disease is threatened by the acceptance of fraudulent therapeutic methods does the medical profession have to draw a line.

The dread of cancer of old has driven desperate patients and their families into the hands of would-be healers and the use of unproven medications. Now that early diagnosis and combination treatment by irradiation therapy, surgery, and chemotherapy has greatly reduced morbidity and mortality from malignancies, this fear should have been replaced by cautious optimism. But two recent incidents of serious quackery do not support such more enlightened attitudes. The first of these incidents was the announcement by two Balkan "healers" about 1952 that they had discovered an anticancer agent in horse serum. They manufactured the product, named it Krebiozen (Krebs is cancer in German), and allied themselves with a prominent physiologist who, in an as yet unexplained delusion, gave the drug respectability. No need to state that Krebiozen was a hoax and did no good.

The second incident was the case of Laetrile. This material was obtained from crushed apricot pits. They were extracted, and the evaporated extract left behind the agent. Chemical studies revealed that it contained a glycoside of mandelonitrile. This known compound can split off highly poisonous hydrogen cyanide, but in very small amounts. Mandelonitrile and its glucoside have no known therapeutic action; hydrogen cyanide is a general cell poison that may have accounted for some of the toxic symptoms caused by Laetrile. Although this information was widely disseminated and supported by a careful study by scientists of the National Institutes of Health (NIH), thousands of deluded cancer patients insisted on taking the "drug." Laetrile was banned in many states, but patients traveled to Mexico, where it remained available. Politicians in several localities were threatened with reprisals if they refused to reintroduce Laetrile. Apart from the deaths directly attributable to the toxicity of Laetrile, patients believing in the power of this agent refused to submit to approved medical methods of cancer treatment and thereby hastened their own demise.

Acquired immune deficiency syndrome (AIDS) is an as-yet incurable slow-onset malignant disease that is transmitted by contact with body fluids of an infected individual. Infection with the causative virus (HIV) may be brought about by sexual contact, by blood transfusion, or by contamination with blood products. The despair, especially among sexually active persons, has led to experimentation with obstruse and indefensible quackery methods of treatment. "Energy soups," mushroom extracts, bee pollen, massage and meditation therapies, herbs to boost the damaged immune system, and even thymus cells in bottles are being offered to desperate victims by fringe practitioners and ruthless profiteers.

A curious invitation to quackery has sprung up in scattered groups of mostly young people who are seeking security in an insecure world by retiring to rural communes. There they try to lead a pioneerlike primitive life. Among their habits is the exclusive consumption of "natural" foods, which they grow themselves or buy in health foods stores. As long as these stores offer an often tasteless diet of nuts and vegetables, one might regard their wares as refreshing variations from prepared, prepackaged, and precooked meals offered by supermarkets. But the shelves of health food stores also hold materials promoted as natural drugs and sources of essential nutrients, minerals and vitamins. They are botanical powders, crystals, oils, and extracts, and some of them are indistinguishable from similar products offered in oriental markets. A number of these products, however, are totally worthless. They must have slipped by the inspection of government agencies that watch over truth in advertising. This would not matter if the customers of these stores would have the facts about such products at their fingertips, but many are uneducated and gullible. Such wasted purchases can only be prevented by more effective consumer protection.

The barrier to dangerous and counterproductive quackery is education of the lay public. Constant reports of suspected cases of quackery, backed by scientific evidence translated into plain English, can dispel superstition and ignorance bordering on voodoo. With a wider emphasis on science in the public schools, the next generation should take a fresh look at beliefs that have come down through the ages, before understanding and searching for the truth had reached the state that we now value. In medicine there is always an outside chance that some natural or synthetic product may turn up as a new and valid therapeutic agent. Until such a claim has been verified by preclinical and approved clinical studies, however, the public should beware and remain skeptical.

The best way to judge the potential therapeutic value of a nonprescription drug preparation is to really read the label specifying its contents. There will usually be some generic name that the lay person may not know. Ask a pharmacist whether the generic product will benefit your condition. If he says it will, take it with confidence but carefully observe dose levels, timing, and other directions on the label. The rest of the list of contents (sugar, solvents, coloring matter, fillers, etc.) may be disregarded.

Appendixes

Appendix A Some Alternative Drug Names

Depending on their origin, history, and manufacture by competing companies, drugs often have alternate proprietary or common names. Most but not all names in the first column are nonproprietary; most of those in the second column are proprietary names, chosen at random and without prejudice. In many cases they represent the major commercial names in the U.S.A. Designations of salts have been omitted.

Nonproprietary Names	*Selected Alternate Names*
Acetaminophen	Tylenol
Acetophenylisatin	Oxyphenisatin acetate
Acetylsalicylic acid	Aspirin
Acrisorcin	Aminacrin
Amantadine	Mydantan
Aminocaproic acid	Amicar
Amobarbital	Amytal
Amphetamine	Benzedrine
Amylocaine	Stovain
Ascorbic Acid	Vitamin C
Bacitracin	Neosporin
Barbital	Veronal
Benzalkonium	Zephiran
Benzethonium chloride	Cepacol
Bialamicol	Camoform
Carbarsone	Amebarsone
Chloramphenicol	Chloromycetin
Chlordantoin	Sporostacin
Chlordiazepoxide	Librium
Chlorguanide	Proguanil
Chlorophenothane	DDT

Chloroquine	Aralen
Chlorothiazide	Diuril
Chlorpromazine	Thorazine
Chlortetracycline	Aureomycin
Cimetidine	Tagamet
Cobalamin	Vitamin B-12
Cycloguanil	Chlorguanide triazine
Cyclophosphamide	Cytoxan
Dapson	Diphenasone
Desipramine	Desmethylimipramine
Dexamethason	Decadrone
Dextroamphetamine	Dexedrine
Diazepam	Valium
Dichlorophen	Parabis
Dicumarol	Dicoumarin
Diethylcarbamazine	Hetrazan
Diethylstilbestrol	DES
Digoxin	Lanoxin
Dimenhydrinate	Dramamine
Diphenadione	Dipaxin
Diphenhydramine	Benadryl
Diphenoxylate	Lomotil
Doxorubicin	Adriamycin
Epinephrine	Adrenaline
Erythromycin	Erythrocin
Estradiol	Progynon
Ethacrynic acid	Edecrine
Ethionamide	Ethimide
Furazepam	Dalmane
Furosemide	Lasix
Glaucarubin	Glarubin
Griseofulvin	Fulvicin
Halazone	Gynamide
Haloperidol	Haldol
Heparin	Panheprin
Hexachlorophene	pH isohex
Hydrochlorthiazide	Hydrodiuril
5-Hydroxytryptamine	Serotonin
Ibuprofen	Motrin, Advil
Imipramine	Tofranil
Indomethacin	Indocin

Iodochlorhydroxyquin	Entero-Vioform
Iproniazid	Marsilid
Isocarboxazid	Marplan
Isoproterenol	Isuprel
Kanamycin	Cantrex
Kaolin	Kaopectate
Leukomycin	Kitasamycin
Lidocaine	Xylocaine
Lincomycin	Lincocin
LSD	Delysid
Lucanthone	Miracil D
Melarsoprol	Mel B
Meperidine	Demerol
Mephobarbital	Mebaral
Meprobamate	Equanil, Miltown
Meralluride	Mercuhydrin
Mercaptopurine	Thiomerin
Methadone	Dolophine
Methamphetamine	Methedrine
Methotrexate	Amethopterin
Methyldopa	Aldomet
Metronidazole	Flagyl
Nialamide	Niamid
Niclosamide	Cestocid
Nitrogen mustard	Mechloramine
Norepinephrine	Noradrenaline
Novobiocin	Panalba
Oleandomycin	Signemycin
Oxine	Quinosol
Oxytetracycline	Terramycin
Pargyline	Eutonyl
Phenelzine	Nardil
Phenobarbital	Luminal
Phenoxymethylpenicillin	Penicillin V
Phenytoin	Dilantin
Prednisolone	Ataraxoid
Prednisone	Arthralgen
Primidone	Mysoline
Procainamide	Pronestyl
Procaine	Novocaine
Progesterone	Progestin

Propranolol	Inderal
Pteroylglutamic acid	Folic acid
Pyrazinamide	Aldinamide
Pyridoxal phosphate	Vitamin B-6
Pyrimethamine	Daraprim
Quinacrine	Atebrin
Reserpine	Serpasil
Retinol	Vitamin A
Riboflavin	Vitamin B-2
Rifampin	Rifampicin
Secobarbital	Seconal
Spiramycin	Sequamycin
Stibocaptate	Astiban
Stibophen	Fuadin
Sulfamethoxazole	Gantanol
Sulfanilamidochrysoidine	Prontosil
Sulfisoxazole	Gantrisin
Sulindac	Clinoril
Suramin	Naphuride
Tetracycline	Achromycin
Theophylline	Choledyl
Thiamine	Vitamin B-1
Thiopental	Pentothal
Thioridazine	Mellaril
Tocopherol	Vitamin E
Tolnaftate	Tinactin
Tranylcypromine	Parnate
Triamterene	Dyazide
Trimethoprim	Syraprim
Tryparsamide	Tryparsone
Tylosin	Tylan
Undecylenic acid	Desenex
Valproic acid	Labazene
Verapamil	Isoproveratril
Vitamins K	Menaquinones
Warfarin	Coumadine

Appendix B
A Glossary of Some Biomedical Terms

Acupuncture The insertion of a needle into parts of the body, blocking the transmission of nerve impulses.

Addiction Dependence on the use of a drug.

Alchemy Chemistry of the Middle Ages; its purpose was to transmute metals into gold and to discover an elixir of youth.

Alkaloid A class of organic chemicals containing nitrogen and usually extracted from plants; some may also occur in animal tissues. Some, but not all, alkaloids are toxic.

Alkylating agent A chemical that combines with proteins and nucleic acids, inactivating these compounds. Used in cancer chemotherapy (q.v.).

Amebiasis Infection caused by the one-celled protozoan *Entamoeba histolytica*.

Analgesic (analgetic) A drug that dampens pain.

Anesthesia Method of making an individual become insensible to pain, changes in temperature, etc., with or without loss of consciousness.

Anesthetic, local A chemical that can numb pain locally without producing unconsciousness.

Angina pectoris Spastic painful condition of the heart muscle, usually due to lack of oxygen.

Anthelmintic A drug used in worm infestation.

Antibiotic Originally a naturally occurring drug produced by microbes and able to halt the spread of certain infectious diseases. Some antibiotics occur in plants; some are manufactured by chemical synthesis. Some are active against cancers; some are used to speed up the growth of livestock. Broad-spectrum antibiotics cure many different diseases.

Antibody A protein produced by the body that can offset the effects of an antigen by reacting with it.

Anticholinergic Drugs that counteract the effects of the neurohormone (q.v.) acetylcholine. Most common activity: relieving the spastic condition of involuntary tissues.

Anticonvulsant Drug that counteracts or prevents convulsions caused by brain diseases, electroshock, or certain chemicals.

Antihistamine (antihistaminic) Drug that counteracts damaging effects of histamine (q.v.) such as allergies, excess stomach acid.

Antihypertensives Drugs that lower elevated blood pressure.

Antimalarials Drugs useful in the chemotherapy (q.v.) of malarias.

Antimetabolite A chemical of a structure related to but not identical with a metabolic biochemical. If it counteracts the effects of the metabolite, it may become a useful drug.

Antipyretic A drug that lowers elevated body temperature.

Antispasmodic A drug that blocks spastic effects of neurohormones, relaxing muscles and preventing excessive secretion from certain glands.

Antitussive A drug that prevents coughing.

Arrhythmia Irregularities in rate of heartbeat.

Arthritis Inflammation of joints. May be a degenerative disease, perhaps related to loss of immune response.

Bactericidal Drugs that kill bacteria.

Bacteriostatic Drugs that slow down or prevent the multiplication ("growth") of bacteria.

Biochemistry The chemistry of substances, processes, and reactions in living organisms, but which can also be studied under laboratory conditions.

Bioisosterism Similarity in molecular shape and binding ability of drugs with similar biological activity.

Biosynthesis Synthesis of a chemical by cells or by a laboratory process analogous to that in living tissue.

Cancer chemotherapy Combatting the spread of malignant cells with drugs.

Cardiac drugs Drugs that regulate functions and contraction (inotropic effect) of the heart.

Cathartics (laxatives) Chemicals that stimulate intestinal peristalsis, relieve constipation.

Chemotherapy Drug treatment of disease-producing foreign cells such as tumor cells, bacteria, viruses, protozoa. Sometimes designates any drug treatment.

Coating, enteric Encapsulating a biologically active chemical in a layer of wax, biodegradable plastic, etc., that will delay and regulate the rate of release of a drug into tissues.

Conditioned avoidance response Behavioral test based on acquired learning.

Convulsion A violent involuntary spasm of the muscles.

Cortex, cerebral Outer layer (gray matter) of the brain.

Cough reflex Physiological response to irritation of bronchial mucous membranes. Involves complex interaction of central and peripheral nerves.

Curare Tarry mixture of substances obtained from the bark of certain tropical vines. Causes paralysis of muscles; is used medicinally to reduce muscular rigidity.

Dendrites Fine branched protrusions of nerve cells involved in transmitting nervous impulses.

Diabetes Hyperglycemia, high blood-sugar levels, resulting from lack of insulin.

Diagnosis Process of deciding the nature of a disease by examination.

Diuretic A drug that increases the secretion and flow of urine. Some diuretics also lower blood pressure.

Drug receptor A protein or nucleic acid that reacts with a drug and initiates a biological effect.

Drug resistance The ability of a cell or organ to ward off the effect of a drug.

Drugs, generic Drugs not (or no longer) the property of a patentee. They can be manufactured and marketed by any suitable agency.

Edema Abnormal accumulation of fluid in cells, tissues, or body cavities resulting in swelling.

Elixir A solution, often an alcoholic tincture, of drugs.

Enkephalins Small-molecular protein neurohormones found in many tissues. They participate in modifying the transmission of painful stimuli.

Enteric coating *See* Coatings, enteric.

Enzyme Protein produced by living cells that has the catalytic ability to regulate rate of biochemical reactions. A few synthetic substances acting like enzymes have become known.

Epilepsy Chronic disease of the central nervous system characterized by convulsions and unconsciousness.

Euphoria A feeling of well-being. Can be induced by certain drugs.

Extrapyramidal symptoms Facial rigidity, tremors, drooling.

FDA U.S. Food and Drug Administration.

Fibrillation, cardiac Heart flutter, irregular beats.

Filariasis Disease caused by nematode worms.

Free radical Unstable fragment of molecules that reacts with oxygen and other reactive chemicals.

Functional disorder Disease affecting a function of an organ, often without an apparent organic change.

Glycosides, cardiac Organic chemicals containing an aglycone and a carbohydrate portion. Some stimulate contractibility of heart muscle. Example: digitalis.

Hallucinogen A drug that can induce mental hallucinations, sometimes psychoses and insanity.

Hibernation, artificial Cooling the body by immersion in cold water or by drugs.

Histamine A neurohormone involved in allergies and some other disease conditions.

Hormone A chemical formed in one organ of the body and carried by the circulation to another tissue, where it exerts a catalytic biological action. Many synthetic hormone analogs are known.

Hyperacidity Excess gastric juice acid.

Hyperglycemia *See* Diabetes.

Hypnotic A sleep-inducing drug; in lower doses, often sedative.

Hypoglycemia Low blood sugar.

Hypophysis *See* Pituitary gland.

Immune system Cellular biochemicals that protect the body against some diseases.

Isotonic Having the same osmotic pressure and salt concentration as blood.

Leishmaniasis Tropical protozoan infection caused by *Leishmaniae*.

Microbiology Science of the chemistry and biology of microbes.

Molecular modification Planned chemical variation of the structure of a prototype drug. Its aim is to improve the therapeutic properties.

Mycobacteria Bacteria naturally encased in a capsule of lipids (fats). They cause slow infections such as leprosy, tuberculosis.

Mycoses Fungus-caused diseases.

Mydriasis Prolonged or excessive dilatation of the pupil of the eye, caused by eye diseases or by a dilating drug.

Neuralgia Superficial or surface pain.

Neurohormone Hormonal chemical secreted at nerve endings and involved in the transmission of nervous impulses.

Neuroleptic A tranquilizing drug; an antipsychotic.

Nonsteroidal antiinflammatory drug A drug useful in arthritis and other inflammatory conditions. Examples: salicylates, indomethacin, ibuprophen, sulindac.

Nutrients, essential Substances in the diet without which deficiency symptoms appear.

Oncogene Cancer inducer.

Opiates Compounds derived from, or similar in action to, potent analgesic opium alkaloids. Many potent synthetic analgesics and euphorics are wrongly called opiates.

Parenteral drugs Administered by injection.

Parkinson's disease Neurological disorder (shaking palsy) accompanied by dopamine deficiency. Exhibits extrapyramidal symptoms (q.v.).

Pathogen An agent or cell that causes disease.

Pathology Branch of medicine studying structural and functional changes caused by disease. Often equated with disease process.

Penicillin A large group of antibacterial antibiotics, some of which are semisynthetic chemicals. Chemically, all are *beta*-lactams.

Peptide A combination of amino acids. A *dipeptide* is a combination of two amino acids; a *polypeptide*, of many amino acids.

Pharmacology The study of the biochemistry, uses, and biological and therapeutic effects of drugs. Not to be confused with pharmacy.

Pharmacopoeia Official compendium listing medicinal drugs, their properties, standards of purity, etc.

"Pill," the (contraceptive) A mixture of estrogen and synthetic progestins that controls menstrual cycles and produces a state of pseudopregnancy, thereby preventing conception.

Pinworm A scalp disease caused by *Oxyuris* worms.

Pituitary gland Also called hypophysis. A small endocrine (hormone-secreting) gland at the base of the brain, affecting metabolism, milk production, body growth, and behavior.

Placebo A preparation containing no medication, but given for its psychological effect.

Prostaglandins A chemically related family of lipid carboxylic acids with twenty carbon atoms, derived from arachidonic acid. They have multiple biological and therapeutic functions.

Psychosis A form of mental illness. A symptom of schizophrenia.

Psychosomatic Physical disorder of the body originating in or aggravated by psychic or emotional activity.

Psychotomimetic A chemical that produces symptoms similar to pathological psychoses. Examples: amphetamine, LSD.

Purines, pyrimidines Hexagonal, ring-shaped chemical structures found in nucleic acids.

Quats Ammonium salts with microbicidal properties.

Recombinant DNA A technique of inserting a foreign gene into the biosynthesis of a DNA, forcing the cell to make the foreign material. Example: Manufacture of human pancreatic insulin by bacteria or yeasts.

Schistosomiasis An infestation caused by schistosome worms that invade body organs.

Schizophrenia A mental disease ("split personality") exhibiting withdrawal, delusions of grandeur and persecution, hallucinations, sometimes psychoses.

Sedative A drug that decreases excitement, irritation, fear.

Sex hormones Chemicals produced by sex organs or occasionally by some other tissues. They determine sexual quality, expression, and behavior and sexual development and processes. Female: estrogens; male: androgens.

Spirochete Slender, spiral-shaped bacteria, some of which cause disease: e.g., syphilis.

Suicide enzyme inhibitor A chemical that reacts as both substrate and inhibitor of an enzyme, using up the enzyme and wasting its catalytic action.

Synapse The minute gap between nerve dendrites (q.v.) across which nerve impulses are transmitted by neurohormones (q.v.).

Teratogen A chemical that causes birth defects.

Tetracyclines A group of broad-spectrum antibiotics with a four-ring structure of atoms.

Thyroid Ductless (endocrine) gland in front and on either side of the windpipe that regulates oxidative processes and growth of the body.

Toxicity Degree of being poisonous.

Trade mark A registered symbol, word, letter, etc., protected by law and used by a manufacturer to distinguish his product from those of competitors.

Trichomoniasis Infectious disease caused by a protozoan microbe called *Trichomonas vaginalis.*

Trypanosome Flagellate protozoans transmitted to humans and other vertebrates by insect vectors; often cause disease.

Trypanosomiasis Diseases caused by trypanosomes, e.g., sleeping sickness, Chagas' disease.

Twilight sleep State of semiconsciousness induced by certain drugs, e.g., scopolamine. It can lessen pain.

Vasoconstrictor A chemical that contracts (narrows) blood vessels.

Virus Complex chemicals consisting of nucleic acids wrapped in a protein capsule of very high molecular weight. Can multiply like animate cells at the expense of its host cell, causing disease.

Vitamins Several chemically different substances that regulate many developmental and bodily functions. Vitamins cannot be biosynthesized in the body, and must be obtained from the diet or from synthetic diet supplements.

X-ray diffraction Method of determining the chemical structure of a compound by measuring the distances between its atoms.

Index